Katrin Hönig

Immune Surveillance in a Novel Transplantation Model Mimicking the Immune Response to Sporadic Cancer

D 188

Bibliographic information published by the Deutsche Nationalbibliothek

The Deutsche Nationalbibliothek lists this publication in the Deutsche
Nationalbibliografie; detailed bibliographic data are available
on the Internet at http://dnb.d-nb.de .

ISBN 978-3-8325-4939-8

Logos Verlag Berlin GmbH
Comeniushof, Gubener Str. 47,
10243 Berlin
Tel.: +49 (0)30 42 85 10 90
Fax: +49 (0)30 42 85 10 92
INTERNET: https://www.logos-verlag.de

Summary

Since decades there is a controversy about the role of the immune system in controlling tumor growth and eliminating transformed cells. For viral induced cancers it has been shown that the immune system is able to surveil tumor growth (Klein and Klein, 1977) but it remains unclear whether spontaneous cancers are recognized by immune cells resulting in a destructive T cell response (Klein et al., 1960; Shankaran et al., 2001; Dunn et al., 2002; Blankenstein and Qin, 2003; Willimsky and Blankenstein, 2005). Because tumorigenesis usually starts from a single transformed cell, it is difficult to simulate sporadic cancer and neoantigen expression by experimental models. Different approaches and mouse models have been used to prove the hypothesis of cancer immune surveillance but almost all of them exhibited limitations in suitability to investigate tumor-specific T cell responses. The aim of this study was to investigate *de novo* T cell responses against a neoantigen expressed by cancer cells under resting conditions. Therefore, a novel transplantation model was established which closely simulated human sporadic cancer development. The question at which time point during tumorigenesis the immune system interacts with nascent cancer cells was answered by this. The cancer cell lines used in this study conditionally expressed SV40 large T (Tag) which is the cancer-driving oncogene and, at the same time, the tumor-specific antigen. Fusion of Tag to firefly luciferase (Luc) enabled visualization of oncogene/antigen expression and tumor growth by non-invasive bioluminescent imaging (BLI). TagLuc expression was tightly regulated by the Tet system and only presence of doxycycline (dox) induced expression of the oncogene/antigen TagLuc and subsequent cancer cell proliferation. In contrast to expectations, temporary inactivation of TagLuc expression by dox withdrawal did not induce cell death in all cancer cells but induced a cell cycle arrest. Moreover, administration of dox to the arrested cancer cells led to re-expression of the oncogene/antigen TagLuc and subsequent cell proliferation. This unique property allowed the inoculation of arrested cancer cells without oncogene/antigen expression and unintended immune responses were avoided by this. After decay of the inoculation-induced acute inflammation, TagLuc was induced under resting conditions and thus, allowed the investigation of neoantigen-specific immune responses as they would occur in human sporadic cancers.

For a closer simulation of early phases of tumorigenesis in which the oncogene/antigen is expressed by only few cells, between 1×10^3 and 1×10^5 arrested cancer cells were inoculated in the conducted experiments of this study. When TagLuc was induced in nascent cancer cells, immunocompetent CM2 mice developed a Tag-specific CD8[+] T cell response and rejected the inoculated cancer cells. Moreover, also old mice developed a destructive, Tag-specific CD8[+] T cell response indicating that immune surveillance of TagLuc expressing cancer cells was not impeded by immunosenescence. In addition, 250-fold lower expression of TagLuc compared to the originally used cell line, also induced Tag-specific CD8[+] T cells suggesting that even though expressed at low amounts, Tag was sufficient to activate CD8[+] T cells under resting conditions. Hence, evidence for immune surveillance of a neoantigen expressed by only few cancer cells in the absence of acute inflammation was demonstrated in this study.

Since sporadic cancers usually develop in the absence of an acute inflammatory environment and mostly do not express positive, T cell co-stimulatory molecules, it is unclear how tumor-specific CD8$^+$ T cells are primed under such conditions. Addressing this question, the role of direct priming was investigated to elucidate potential mechanisms of CD8$^+$ T cell activation in the presented model. Adoptive transfer experiments revealed that priming of naïve Tag-specific CD8$^+$ T cells was independent of CD4$^+$ T cell help and occurred in the absence of cross-presentation. Although the missing opportunity to cross-present TagLuc delayed the activation of naïve CD8$^+$ T cells, cancer cells were rejected ultimately in an MHC-mismatched host. These results imply the relevance of direct priming for the induction of cytotoxic T cell responses against neoantigens expressed by sporadic cancer.

In summary, results obtained in this study strongly argue for immune surveillance of nascent cancer cells. This study demonstrates for the first time that neoantigen-specific CD8$^+$ T cells were induced in the absence of acute inflammation and CD8$^+$ T cells were primed directly by cancer cells. However, Tag represents a particular type of tumor antigens since it comprises multiple epitopes recognized by T cells, thus increasing the probability of eliciting an immune response. In future studies, the presented model can be utilized to investigate immune surveillance against neoantigens caused by a single point mutation as they are found in the majority of human sporadic cancers. Will immunity still be there?

Zusammenfassung

Seit Beginn des 20. Jahrhunderts wird die Rolle des Immunsystems bei der Überwachung des Tumorwachstums und der Elimination transformierter Zellen kontrovers diskutiert. Bei durch Viren induzierten Tumoren wurde bereits gezeigt, dass das Immunsystem Tumorwachstum kontrollieren kann (Klein and Klein, 1977). Bei spontanen Tumoren ist jedoch unklar, ob diese durch Immunzellen erkannt werden und es zu einer destruktiven Immunantwort kommt (Klein et al., 1960; Shankaran et al., 2001; Dunn et al., 2002; Blankenstein and Qin, 2003; Willimsky and Blankenstein, 2005). Weil es schwierig ist, die Entstehung sporadischer Tumoren mit experimentellen Modellen zu simulieren, sind viele bisher verwendete Modelle nur begrenzt geeignet Tumorantigen-spezifische T-Zell-Antworten zu untersuchen. Ziel der vorliegenden Arbeit war es, *de novo* T-Zell-Antworten gegen ein Neoantigen, welches nicht unter akuten, entzündlichen Bedingungen von Krebszellen exprimiert wird, in einem dazu neu entwickelten Transplantationsmodell zu untersuchen. Mittels Simulation der sporadischen Tumorentstehung wurde die Frage beantwortet, zu welchem Zeitpunkt das Immunsystem mit auftretenden Krebszellen interagiert. Das neu etablierte Transplantationsmodell ermöglichte die Expression eines Neoantigens in Krebszellen ohne die sonst mit einer Transplantation einhergehenden akuten Entzündung. Die verwendeten Krebszelllinien exprimierten konditionell SV40 large T (Tag) als krebsantreibendes Onkogen, welches gleichzeitig auch als Tumorantigen fungiert. Durch dessen Fusion mit Luziferase (Luc) konnte sowohl die Onkogen-/Antigenexpression als auch das Tumorwachstum durch nicht-invasives Biolumineszenzimaging (BLI) visualisiert werden. TagLuc-Expression in den Krebszellen wurde durch das Tet-System eng reguliert und das Onkogen/Antigen wurde nur in Anwesenheit von Doxycyclin (Dox) induziert. Interessanterweise führte eine temporäre, durch Dox-Entzug verursachte Inaktivierung von TagLuc nicht zum Absterben aller Zellen, sondern zu einem Zellzyklusarrest. TagLuc konnte später durch erneute Doxgabe wieder induziert werden, woraufhin die überlebenden Krebszellen proliferierten. Diese einzigartige Fähigkeit erlaubte die Inokulation von arretierten Krebszellen, die kein Onkogen/Antigen exprimieren, wodurch eine unerwünschte Erkennung durch das Immunsystem vermieden wurde. Nach Abklingen der durch Inokulation verursachten, akuten Entzündung, wurde TagLuc induziert, um neoantigenspezifische Immunantworten unter Bedingungen, wie sie bei sporadischen Tumoren des Menschen vorkommen, zu untersuchen.

Um eine frühe Phase der Tumorentstehung zu simulieren, in der das Onkogen/Antigen nur in wenigen Zellen anstatt in einem etablierten Tumor exprimiert ist, wurden zwischen 1×10^3 und 1×10^5 Krebszellen inokuliert. Wenn TagLuc in ruhenden Krebszellen induziert wurde, entwickelten immunkompetente CM2-Mäuse eine Tag-spezifische CD8$^+$ T-Zell-Antwort und stießen die inokulierten Krebszellen ab. Diese Immunantwort konnte auch bei alten Mäusen beobachtet werden. Dieses Ergebnis impliziert, dass die Immunüberwachung von TagLuc-exprimierenden Krebszellen nicht durch Immunseneszenz verhindert wurde. Ebenso reichte eine um das 250-fache geringere TagLuc-Expression in Krebszellen aus, um CD8$^+$ T-Zellen unter nicht-akutentzündlichen Bedingungen zu aktivieren. Damit wurde in der vorliegenden Arbeit gezeigt, dass die Immunüberwachung von Neoantigenexprimierenden Krebszellen auch in frühen Phasen der Tumorentstehung stattfindet und zu einer destruktiven CD8$^+$ T-Zell-Antwort führt.

Sporadische Tumoren entwickeln sich für gewöhnlich in Abwesenheit von akuter Entzündung und exprimieren nur selten positive, kostimulatorische Moleküle. Deshalb ist es unklar, wie tumorspezifische CD8$^+$ T-Zellen unter diesen Bedingungen aktiviert werden. Die Rolle der direkten T-Zell-Aktivierung durch Krebszellen wurde mittels adoptiver Zelltransferexperimente untersucht. Diese Experimente zeigten, dass naive, Tag-spezifische CD8$^+$ T-Zellen unabhängig von CD4$^+$ T-Zell-Hilfe und ohne Antigen-Kreuzpräsentation durch andere Immunzellen aktiviert wurden. Obwohl die fehlende Möglichkeit der Antigen-Kreuzpräsentation in Haupthistokompatibilitätskomplex (MHC, major histocompatibility complex) -inkompatiblen Rezipienten zu einer verzögerten Aktivierung von naiven CD8$^+$ T-Zellen führte, wurden die Krebszellen letztendlich abgestoßen. Diese Ergebnisse implizieren die Relevanz der direkten CD8$^+$ T-Zell-Aktivierung bei Immunantworten gegen Neoantigen-exprimierende, sporadische Tumoren.

Zusammengefasst, liefert die vorliegende Arbeit starke Beweise dafür, dass Immunüberwachung von aufkommenden Krebszellen existiert. Neoantigen-spezifische CD8$^+$ T-Zellen wurden unter nicht-akut-entzündlichen Bedingungen induziert und diese nachweislich direkt durch Krebszellen aktiviert. Das in dieser Studie untersuchte Antigen Tag repräsentiert jedoch eine besondere Gruppe von Tumorantigen. Es besitzt mehrere Epitope, die von T-Zellen erkannt werden und dadurch *per se* mit höherer Wahrscheinlichkeit eine Immunantwort hervorrufen können. Das beschriebene Modell kann zukünftig eingesetzt werden, um die Immunüberwachung von Krebszellen, die ein durch eine Punktmutation verursachtes Neoantigen exprimieren, zu untersuchen. Wird es auch da Immunität geben?

Table of Contents

1 Introduction

1.1 The immune system

The function of the immune system is to discriminate non-self pathogens from self tissues (Burnet, 1961). For survival of multicellular organisms, it is important to recognize harmful pathogens, e.g. viruses and bacteria, and to protect against diseases or potentially damaging threats and hence, ensure functional integrity of the organism. The division of the immune system into innate and adaptive immunity has helped to understand the immune response, but it is essential to consider that the immune system functions as one unit rather than as separate entities. Cells of the innate immunity, e.g. macrophages and natural killer (NK) cells act as a first line defense against pathogens. They express pattern recognition receptors, e.g. toll-like receptors, recognizing conserved molecular patterns associated with microbes and pathogens (Janeway and Medzhitov, 2002). Subsequent signaling leads to activation of innate and adaptive immunity through synthesized molecules, e.g. cytokines. The defense mechanisms of the innate immunity are effective in combating many pathogens, but the receptor repertoire of innate immune cells is limited and invariant. Different from the unspecific antigen recognition by the innate immune system, the adaptive immune system comprises B and T cells with a high receptor diversity and thus enables specific recognition of antigens by exhibiting more precise mechanisms (Iwasaki and Medzhitov, 2015).

Achieving immunity to cancer is a challenging task for the immune system because cancer is not an exogenous pathogen but arises from normal host cells. Therefore, assignment of cancer cells to self or non-self is difficult because cancer antigens recognized by the immune system are self or mutated self molecules.

1.2 The concept of immune surveillance theory

It was Paul Ehrlich, who first came up with the idea that a protective mechanism may exist, which protects the organism from malignancies that otherwise would arise with great frequencies (Ehrlich, 1909). He distinguished between immunological responses and cellular resistance, that prevent malignant transformation of somatic cells. However, this hypothesis was not proven experimentally because adequate experimental systems and detailed knowledge about cellular immunity were lacking at this time. With the developing knowledge about cellular immunology in the 1950s, the concept of immune surveillance came into focus of scientists' interest, which resulted in the postulation of the immune surveillance hypothesis by Burnet and Thomas (Burnet, 1957; Thomas, 1959). They both independently proposed that complex organisms must possess a defense system that recognizes and eliminates nascent tumor cells. They argued that tissues in which cells undergo numerous proliferation cycles, have a great capability for acquiring genetic mutations that results in transformation of cells and tumorigenesis. Since then, many efforts have been made to prove or disprove the hypothesis, that the adaptive immune system plays a role in eliminating cancer cells.

The immune system evolved to distinguish self from non-self and thereby protects the organism from infections with viruses, bacteria or other pathogens. Whether the immune system is involved in protection of the organism from cancer is the subject of hot debates. Because a cancerous cell originates from a 'self' somatic or, in rarer cases, a germline cell, its recognition as 'non-self' by immune cells implies the expression of proteins that are different from those expressed by normal cells. Prehn and Main published first experimental evidence for immunity against carcinogen-induced autochthonous tumors in mice. They demonstrated that each tumor induced a specific immune response, which suggests the existence of unique molecules that are recognized as tumor-specific antigens (Prehn and Main, 1957). Later, Klein et al. showed that even progressing tumors can elicit an immune response: If the primary tumor was surgically removed and cultured, mice rejected a challenge with cells from the same tumor. However, this immune response was only observed if the host was immunized with the same, previously irradiated tumor cells prior to tumor challenge. Without prior immunization, mice were unable to reject and tumors progressed (Klein et al., 1960). One has to note that the identification of such tumor-specific rejection antigens remained missing in these studies.

To prove the concept of cancer immune surveillance, many experiments have been conducted in hosts with a compromised immune system. The susceptibility to tumors is supposed to be much higher in hosts lacking cells from the adaptive immune system compared to hosts with an intact immune system. In fact, this was shown for approaches using virus-induced tumors or chemically induced tumors and mice that underwent neonatal thymectomy (Grant and Miller, 1965; Nomoto and Takeya, 1969; Burstein and Law, 1971). But it was on debate, whether these findings could be ascribed to defective control of the viral infection in transformed cells or to an impaired immune response. With discovery of the mutant 'nude' mouse which has no functional thymus and thus, has a lack of T cells and deficits in adaptive immunity, a better mouse model was available to test the cancer immune surveillance hypothesis (Flanagan, 1966). Stutman showed clearly that neither spontaneous nor carcinogen-induced tumors occurred with shorter latencies or higher frequencies in T cell-deficient nude mice compared to immunocompetent wildtype mice (Stutman, 1974). It has to be mentioned that wildtype mice used as controls in this study were littermates from the same breeding. As a consequence, environmental differences caused by a separate breeding of control mice and their effect on potential immune responses were excluded.

For virus-induced tumors, Klein et al. demonstrated that immune surveillance is indeed effective in rejecting virus-transformed cells (Klein and Klein, 1977). Tumor resistance is rather due to immune responses against virally determined cell antigens than to the viral infection *per se* (Schreiber, 2012b). The immune surveillance hypothesis vanished in oblivion until novel gene-engineering technologies have been developed in the 1990s. New techniques allowed the development of mouse models with a molecularly defined immunodeficiency. These included Rag$^{-/-}$ mice, lacking T, B and NKT cells; mice lacking important immune cytokines or their receptors, e.g. interferon gamma (IFN-γ); mice lacking signaling pathways involved immune responses, e.g. STAT1 (signal transducer and activator of transcription 1); and mice lacking important immune cell effector functions, e.g. perforin$^{-/-}$ mice with absent cytotoxic T and NK cell function. Comparing the susceptibility to carcinogen 3-methylcholanthrene (MCA)-induced tumorigenesis in different immunodeficient mice to wildtype mice, revealed inconsistent findings regarding immune surveillance: lack of perforin (van den Broek et al., 1996) or IFN-γ (Kaplan et al., 1998) resulted in increased tumor incidence, which was confirmed by some groups (Smyth et al., 1999; Shankaran et al., 2001) but not by others (Noguchi et al., 1996; Qin and Blankenstein, 2004; Kammertoens et al., 2012). One reason that incidence for MCA-induced cancers in Rag$^{-/-}$ mice is not reproducible is that most of the researchers did not use controls at all (van den Broek et al., 1996) or they did not use littermates as adequate control of their experiments. For example, Smyth and colleagues used for their experiments in perforin$^{-/-}$ mice historical controls instead of littermates from the same breeding (Smyth et al., 1999). Further explanations for these controversial findings were pointed out by Schreiber and Podack (Schreiber and Podack, 2009): they demonstrate differences in critical parameters, e.g. MCA dose, route of injection, mouse strain, housing conditions; and differences in the presentation of data. Some investigators showed tumor growth curves whereas others reported percentage of tumor free mice regardless of a precise definition of the term 'tumor free'. Taken together, all these differences impact the reported tumor incidence upon MCA administration and thereby results cannot be compared directly. Interestingly, Briesemeister et al. demonstrated clearly that serum cytokine levels are significantly different between wildtype mice and mice carrying either one or two alleles of a targeted mutation. This suggests that mice from breeding colonies with a targeted mutation have an altered base-line inflammatory response (Briesemeister et al., 2012). The results of this study underline the importance of using control littermates instead of control mice from a separate breeding and imply that different tumor incidences observed in experiments with MCA can be mainly attributed to the use of inappropriate controls.

Besides the finding by Shankaran et al. that IFN-γ and lymphocytes protect against MCA-induced tumors, they demonstrated for the first time that tumors grown in immunodeficient mice were more immunogenic than tumors raised in immunocompetent mice. This result strengthened the original hypothesis of immune surveillance by Burnet and Thomas, which was extended to the hypothesis of immunoediting by Dunn and colleagues. The concept of immunoediting comprises three phases, termed elimination, equilibrium and escape. Dunn et al. explained that transformed cells are initially recognized and destroyed by immune cells. But occasionally, a population of transformed cells may resist elimination. This cancer cell population is supposed to be less immunogenic, may finally escape by different mechanisms and is not capable of eliciting an immune response (Dunn et al., 2002). Nevertheless, profound evidence for this hypothesis is missing because T cells in a primary host have never been examined in those studies.

1.3 Immune surveillance of human cancer

The role of the immune system in preventing tumor growth in humans was first studied in the 1980s and 1990s by analyzing clinical data from solid organ and bone marrow transplant recipients and HIV patients. The frequency of Kaposi's sarcoma was found to be highly increased in those immunocompromised individuals (Haverkos and Drotman, 1985; Farge, 1993). However, that data merely demonstrate the role of the immune system in controlling virally induced tumors, because a herpesvirus (HHV-8) is responsible for Kaposi's sarcoma. Further types of cancer with increased incidences in immunosuppressed individuals are Epstein-Barr virus (EBV) -induced B cell lymphoma (Oertel and Riess, 2002) and Hodgkin lymphoma, human papilloma virus (HPV) -induced cervical, anal, vulvar, oral and skin cancer or hepatitis B and C virus-induced hepatocellular carcinoma (Grulich et al., 2007).

Evidence of immune surveillance in human cancer was also found in tumors with a certain genetic instability, referred to as microsatellite instability (MSI). Tumors with MSI have defects in DNA mismatch repair mechanisms, which leads to the duplication or deletion of short repeated DNA sequences known as microsatellites. In genetically unstable colorectal cancer, MSI was associated with high amounts of activated cytotoxic lymphocytes hinting at a role of the immune system in controlling tumor growth (Guidoboni et al., 2001). Further, the infiltration with activated T cells and other lymphocytes in colorectal cancer with a high degree of MSI (MSI-H) indicates a local immune response (Dolcetti et al., 1999). However, antigen specificity of tumor-infiltrating T cells is largely unknown. A new report by Simoni et al. shows that the majority of tumor-infiltrating CD8$^+$ T cells recognized epitopes that were unrelated to the cancer, e.g. viral antigens (Simoni et al., 2018) The high mutation rate in MSI-H tumors has been shown to generate *de novo* tumor antigens that can be recognized by the adaptive immune system including CD8$^+$ T cells (Saeterdal et al., 2001; Ishikawa et al., 2003). Ishikawa analyzed potential neoepitopes by SEREX (serological identification of antigens by recombinant expression cloning). Using this technique, a frameshift mutation in the coding region of CDX2 was detected and they also found antibodies against the corresponding antigen in a cancer patient. However, development of specific antibodies did not prevent tumor outgrowth in this patient (Ishikawa et al., 2003). Saeterdal et al. identified a frameshift mutation in the transforming growth factor beta receptor type II (TGF β RII) gene. This mutation was recognized by a cytotoxic T lymphocyte (CTL) clone derived from a healthy donor, but if the same mutation would have been recognized by patient's CTLs remains unclear (Saeterdal et al., 2001). The association of MSI-H in tumors and strong lymphocyte infiltration was also found in other cancer types, e.g. non-medullary gastric cancer (Lu et al., 2004) and resectable pancreatic cancer (Nakata et al., 2002).

Tumor infiltrating lymphocytes (TILs) might be another evidence for the immunoediting theory. Infiltration of tumors by T cells, but also NK and NKT cells, has been associated with an improved prognosis for different tumors, e.g. melanoma (Clemente et al., 1996), ovarian cancer (Zhang et al., 2003) and colorectal cancer (Galon et al., 2006). In general, most data obtained from TIL studies are suggestive because T cell specificities are not known and thus, it is questionable if they resemble immune surveillance as postulated by Burnet and Thomas (Burnet, 1957; Thomas, 1959). Since methods for identification of mutations in tumors emerged during the last decade, it is now possible to analyze individual patient's tumor exome and detect somatic mutations that are recognized by autologous tumor infiltrating T cells. In 2016, the group of Steven A. Rosenberg screened peripheral blood of melanoma patients and identified CD8$^+$ T cells that recognize unique, patient-specific neo-antigens. This demonstrated that immunoediting as postulated by Dunn and colleagues (Dunn et al., 2004) did not occur during melanoma development. Although the function of those neoantigen-specific CD8$^+$ T cells remained unclear, the results from this study suggest that they were dysfunctional because the melanoma developed despite the presence of those CD8$^+$ T cells (Gros et al., 2016).

However, most of the information about human anti-tumor immune responses was obtained from studies with cancer patients and thus, only late phases of tumorigenesis were investigated. Furthermore, except for virus-induced cancers, all human studies only exhibit correlations between cancer and T cell occurrence. It remains unclear at which time during tumorigenesis the immune system initially interacts with cancer cells and whether an observed anti-tumor response would ever be a tumor rejection response.

1.4   Presentation of tumor antigens to T cells

T cells harbor specific T cell receptors (TCRs) that recognize peptides bound to major histocompatibility complex (MHC) molecules expressed on the surface of each cell. TCRs of CD8$^+$ T cells are restricted to MHC class I molecules which are located on the cell surface of all nucleated cells, whereas TCRs of CD4$^+$ T cells are restricted to MHC class II molecules, which are expressed exclusively on professional antigen-presenting cells (APCs), e.g. DCs, macrophages and B cells. Hence, the recognition of tumor antigens by CD8$^+$ T cells requires their presentation on MHC class I molecules either by cancer cells themselves or by other host cells (Murphy et al., 2008a). Before loading of antigens onto MHC class I molecules, a complex process of antigen degradation into peptide fragments takes place in cytosolic and nuclear proteasomes (Townsend and Bodmer, 1989; Yewdell and Bennink, 1992). The resulting peptides mostly comprise lengths between 8 and 10 amino acids and are translocated from the cytoplasm to the endoplasmic reticulum (ER) by the transport protein TAP (transporter associated with antigen presentation) (Kleijmeer et al., 1992; Yewdell et al., 1993). Finally, the MHC class I molecule/peptide complexes are assembled in the ER and released for presentation on the cell surface (Pamer and Cresswell, 1998).

It is believed that the differentiation of a naïve CD8$^+$ T cell into a cytotoxic T cell is not solely dependent on the so-called first signal, which is characterized by direct peptide/MHC and TCR interactions. In addition, the engagement of the co-stimulatory receptor CD28 on T cells by ligands of the B7 family members expressed on professional APCs provides a further necessary signal for differentiation of cytotoxic T cells (Linsley et al., 1991). Chemokines and cytokines, especially IL-12, secreted by APCs provide an additional signal, which leads to a fully activated effector CD8$^+$ T cell that can kill antigen-presenting tumor cells by induction of apoptosis (Murphy et al., 2008b). It is postulated that antigen recognition in the absence of the second signal – as it probably occurs in peripheral tissues and thus in most solid tumors – renders T cells non-reactive or induces deletion (Bretscher and Cohn, 1970; Schwartz, 1990; Matzinger, 1994). However, experiments in mice deficient for the co-stimulatory receptor CD28 showed that persistent presence of the antigen and subsequent TCR-p/MHC interaction generates a functional T cell response *in vivo* without a co-stimulatory signal (Kündig et al., 1996). This finding was supported by a study from Pardigon et al., in which naïve CD8$^+$ T cells were fully activated by the presence of TCR-peptide/MHC interaction alone. However, co-stimulation lowered the activation threshold of T cells (Pardigon et al., 1998). In conclusion, the importance of co-stimulation in inducing functional T cell responses is not completely understood. Nevertheless, the importance of antigen presentation in priming of naïve T cells is beyond question. There are two pathways involved in activation of tumor antigen-specific CD8$^+$ T cells: Direct priming by tumor antigens presented through MHC class I molecules expressed on cancer cells themselves (Fig. 1.1a) or cross-priming by tumor antigens that were taken up, loaded onto MHC class I molecules and presented to CD8$^+$ T cells by professional APCs (Fig. 1.1b). It is generally accepted that naive CD8$^+$ T cells are most efficiently primed by APCs, mainly DCs, in secondary lymphoid organs, e.g. tumor-draining lymph nodes. Thereto, MHC class I-restricted tumor antigens need to be cross-presented by APCs. Consequently, this process is called cross-presentation (Bevan, 1976), which is characterized by a selective transport of internalized antigens to the cytosol to enter the antigen-processing machinery and the MHC class I antigen-presenting pathway (Rodriguez et al., 1999) (Fig. 1.1b). There is convincing evidence that tumor antigens are efficiently cross-presented *in vivo* (Huang et al., 1994; Boonman et al., 2004; van Mierlo et al., 2004). However, in a process called direct presentation antigens can be presented directly to naïve CD8$^+$ T cells by tumor cells themselves. Albeit, the majority of immunologists believe this mechanism is inherently defective because most tumors do not express co-stimulatory molecules to activate T cells (Chen et al., 1993) (Fig. 1.1a). However, the group of Zinkernagel demonstrated that direct priming of T cells by tumor cells in the draining lymph nodes induces a cytotoxic T cell response if sufficient tumor cells reach secondary lymphatic organs early and for long enough duration (Ochsenbein et al., 2001). Experiments performed with tumor cells expressing neoantigens in TAP-deficient mice supported the results of Zinkernagel and clearly showed that MHC class I-proficient tumors cells that are present in the draining lymph nodes can induce antigen-specific T cell responses (Wolkers et al., 2001).

Considering the contradicting results in scientific literature, it remained yet unclear how naïve CD8$^+$ T cells are activated and whether direct or cross-priming takes place in the context of tumor-specific immune responses. The mode of T cell activation may depend on several factors, such as antigen expression, antigen/MHC complex expression and the accessibility of an antigen to the pathway of cross presentation. The latter is discussed for the model antigen gp33 which appears to be resistant to cross-presentation (Ochsenbein et al., 2001; discussed in Heath et al., 2004).

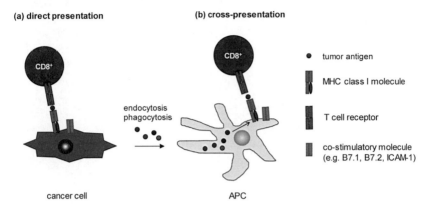

Figure 1.1 Priming of tumor-reactive CD8⁺ T cells
(a) Direct presentation is characterized by cancer cells displaying processed antigenic peptides in a complex with MHC class I molecules on their surface thereby activating CD8⁺ T cells. This requires additional stimulation of CD8⁺ T cells by co-stimulatory molecules expressed on the cancer cells. **(b)** Cross-presentation is characterized by APCs, e.g. dendritic cells, acquiring tumor antigens obtained from cancer cells through endocytosis or phagocytosis. Those antigens are loaded – with or without processing – onto MHC class I molecules for presentation to CD8⁺ T cells. Likewise, additional stimulation through co-stimulatory molecules is required for full activation of the T cells. Figure modified from (You et al., 2017).

1.5 Tumor antigens

Tumor antigens are any molecules expressed by cancer cells that can be detected by T cells (Schreiber, 2012a). Thus, they play an important role in diagnosis and treatment of cancer. Only the presence of tumor antigens make cancer accessible for anti-tumor immune responses and targeted immunotherapies (Blankenstein et al., 2012).

Tumor antigens can be divided into two main classes: tumor-specific and self-antigens. Tumor-specific antigens arise from mutations and are usually expressed exclusively by tumor cells (Coulie et al., 1995; Monach et al., 1995; Wolfel et al., 1995). These antigens are often referred to as neoantigens and can be shared by several cancers if the same mutation occurs (Takahashi et al., 1989; Kessler et al., 2006), which is, by comparison, relatively rare. Although the unique expression of tumor-specific antigens theoretically eases the recognition of cancer cells as non-self, which is an important criterion for eliciting anti-tumor responses, only few of them were demonstrated to be immunogenic (e.g. Robbins et al., 2013). In contrast to tumor-specific antigens, self-antigens are non-mutated and encoded in the genome of all cells but expressed predominantly or at high levels by cancer cells (Offringa, 2009). Because expression of these antigens is not cancer-specific, they are often referred to as tumor-associated antigens. Tumor-associated antigens can be categorized into different subgroups: (I) Overexpressed proteins, such as HER2/neu found in breast and ovarian cancer (Coussens et al., 1985) and Wilms' tumor protein 1 (WT-1) found in leukemia (Call et al., 1990) are expressed in normal tissues but at much higher levels on cancer cells. (II) Differentiation antigens, such as CD19 expressed on B cells (Uckun et al., 1988) or gp-100 and MART-1 expressed on melanocytes (Bakker et al., 1994; Kawakami et al., 1994), are lineage-specific and thus, tumors expressing these antigens originate from the same tissues. (III) Cancer-testis antigens, such as members of the MAGE family (Traversari et al., 1992; Simpson et al., 2005), are reactivated proteins encoded by genes specific for germ cells and are usually expressed by spermatocytes in the testis (Scanlan et al., 2002). (IV) Tumor antigens caused by altered glycosylation, such as COSMC (Schietinger et al., 2006) or Tn (Moreau et al., 1957), are proteins that show aberrant glycosylation or overexpression of certain carbohydrates. All tumor-associated antigens have in common that potential adaptive immune responses should be directed against cancer cells, but not to normal cells expressing those antigens. However, the presentation of tumor-associated antigens — which are at the same time tissue-specific self-antigens — by thymic epithelial cells induces central T cell tolerance and thus, effective endogenous anti-tumor responses are limited (Gotter et al., 2004; Anderson and Su, 2011).

A special type of tumor-specific antigens are viral antigens which comprise of oncoviral proteins encoded by viral genes and not by host genes.

1.6 Relevance of existing cancer models to study tumor-specific T cell responses and immune surveillance

Various models exist to investigate the immune response to cancer. However, the choice of an appropriate model strongly depends on the question asked. In order to answer the century-old question, if the immune system protects us from cancer, different approaches and mouse models have been used. Most, if not all, of these models exhibited limitations regarding suitability to analyze tumor-specific T cell responses in – preferentially– the primary, tumor-bearing host. One example is the widely used experimental approach to chemically induce sarcomas by application of MCA. Various research groups compared frequencies of MCA-induced tumors in immunocompetent and immunodeficient hosts and published contradicting findings regarding the role of the immune system in prevention of tumor growth (Klein et al., 1960; Stutman, 1974; Kaplan et al., 1998; Kammertoens et al., 2012). However, analysis of tumor-specific immune responses in the MCA model is not possible because the tumor antigens are usually not known and thus, a mechanism how immune surveillance takes place cannot be explored. A study published by Matsushita et al., applied cancer-exome analysis of an MCA-induced sarcoma from an immunodeficient Rag$^{-/-}$ mouse and identified a potential rejection antigen (Matsushita et al., 2012). This has also been shown already many years before by demonstrating that UV light-induced tumors harbor tumor-specific mutant genes encoding for tumor-specific antigens (Kripke, 1974; Ward et al., 1989). Nevertheless, potential tumor-specific T cell responses against those antigens were not analyzed in the primary host. Consequently, it remained unclear if an antigen-specific T cell response observed upon transplantation into an immunocompetent host would ever be destructive in a setting resembling sporadic tumor formation. Moreover, it is important to consider that carcinogen-induced tumors, e.g. induced by MCA or UV light, are expected to harbor high numbers of mutations which are rarely found in human sporadic cancers (Khong and Restifo, 2002). The mutational burden of most human cancers is rather low, ranging between less than one mutation per mega base for several leukemias and up to 10 mutations per mega base for some solid cancers, e.g. melanoma and lung cancer (Alexandrov et al., 2013). In addition, susceptibility to chemical carcinogenesis is influenced by unspecific inflammatory responses, which may differ between immunocompetent and immunodeficient hosts but also between wildtype and targeted mutation breeding colonies (Briesemeister et al., 2012).

Another approach to elucidate the role of the immune system during tumor formation is the transplantation of cancer cells or tumors. In these models, tumors usually grow fast and thereby reflect the progression but not early development of a sporadic tumor. However, the major problem of transplanted tumor models is their artificial character. Usually a high number of already transformed tumor cells is injected which results in acute inflammation at the inoculation site (Schreiber et al., 2006). The resulting infiltration of immune cells can lead to unintended immune responses. Moreover, inoculation is accompanied by increased tumor cell death and as a result, high antigen amounts are released to the environment. Presentation of these tumor antigens to T cells that randomly circulate to local lymph nodes, can lead to an unintended tumor cell rejection that would not occur in the absence of acute inflammation. Development and progression of (sporadic) cancer is shown to require a chronic but not acute inflammatory environment (Mantovani et al., 2008). Thus, the acute inflammation accompanying tumor cell transplantation poorly reflects a situation found in early tumorigenesis of sporadic cancers. Consequently, anti-tumor T cell responses observed upon tumor transplantation might be mainly caused by experimental artifacts.

Genetically engineered mouse models (GEMMs) can overcome the problems caused by tumor transplantation by simulating sporadic tumor formation in the absence of inflammation and in the natural tumor microenvironment. In those models, transgenic oncogene expression is controlled by tissue-specific or ubiquitous promoters and its induction leads to cellular transformation and tumorigenesis. If in addition a tumor-specific antigen is expressed by the arising tumor, GEMMs enable the analysis of specific adaptive immune responses. Nevertheless, modeling of sporadic tumor formation also remains difficult with GEMMs. One problem is that (tumor) antigen expression in normal tissues likely modifies T cell responses and additionally, thymic deletion of antigen-specific T cells typically prevents the study of endogenous T cell responses to tumors. For example, this was observed in mouse models of prostate cancer (Savage et al., 2008) and pancreatic cancer (Speiser et al., 1997; Lyman et al., 2004). Since transgenic mouse tumor models without conditional oncogene expression base on sporadic tumor-initiating events that can vary widely between tumors, but also between different mice, it is difficult to follow the dynamics of T cell responses over time (Frese and Tuveson, 2007). In contrast, GEMMs of many human cancers aim to recapitulate tumor progression from early lesions to metastasis by spatiotemporally control of the tumor onset. Using those models, arising cancer exerts the genetic and histopathologic features found in human cancer and allows to study the interaction between tumors and the immune system. But a major problem of these GEMMs is that the conditional expression of onco-genes driven by ubiquitous or tissue-specific promoters almost always leads to multiple tu-mors. Further, an artificially high number of cells is transformed simultaneously. In conse-quence, GEMMs do not accurately resemble human cancer development, which usually originates from one transformed cell. These highly advanced tumor models also show other limitations in respect to sporadic tumor formation. For example, Willimsky and Blanken-stein describe a mouse tumor model in which the oncogene SV40 T antigen (Tag) is dormant because of a loxP site-flanked stop cassette that separates the oncogene from the promoter. Only excision of the stop cassette by an active Cre recombinase lead to induction of Tag expression. However, they observed a stop cassette deletion due to rare, stochastic events and sporadic tumors developed after long latency in LoxP-Tag mice. Despite an initial in-duction of tumor-specific T cells, tumors progressed. This may be caused by an uncontrol-lable leakiness of the transgene at more than one site of the body, which lead to anergic T cells in this model (Willimsky and Blankenstein, 2005). In 2011, Anders et al. established a mouse model combining a tissue-specific Cre recombinase with conditionally regulated ex-pression of a fusion protein consisting of SV40 large T antigen (Tag) and firefly luciferase (Fluc). Additionally, expression of TagLuc is prevented by a loxP site-flanked stop cassette separating the promoter from the oncogene TagLuc. Only Cre recombinase-mediated dele-tion of the stop cassette and concurrent doxycycline (dox)-induced activation of a transacti-vator (CAG-rtTA) should have led to TagLuc expression and consequent tumor develop-ment. But also, in this model a sporadic tumor developed independent of Cre recombination. More than 1 year after dox-mediated TagLuc induction, a gastric carcinoma was isolated from a $TRE^{loxP}stop^{loxP}TagLuc^{+/-}/CAG-rtTA^{+/-}$ mouse (Anders et al., 2011a). Both examples imply the importance of tightly controlled oncogene expression that is essential to exclude tumor specific tolerance induced by leakiness of transgene expression. Further, tumors in both models developed after a long latency which requires time-consuming and expensive experiments. In addition, the oncogene in such GEMMs is induced in millions of cells in the respective tissue, which does not reflect a physiological situation during formation of spo-radic tumors.

In an autochthonous lung cancer model published by DuPage et al., endogenous T cell re-sponses against antigens expressed by lung tumors upon lentiviral delivery were observed. Nevertheless, the use of lentiviral vectors has important limitations since antigen expression cannot be completely restricted to tumor cells and the viral infection may alter the outcome of an anti-tumor immune response. Further, tumors expressed ovalbumin, an artificial model antigen which is unlikely to be expressed by human sporadic cancers (DuPage et al., 2011). Moreover, Willimsky et al. showed that adenoviral induction of Tag as a cancer-driving oncogene in hepatocytes initiated −besides Tag-specific $CD8^+$ T cells− a virus-specific $CD8^+$ T cell response that led to clearance of the infected cells (Willimsky et al., 2013). Both ex-amples demonstrate that models using viral vectors to activate tumor antigen expression do not reflect sporadic tumor formation and potential immune surveillance because it cannot be excluded that expression of viral antigens induces rejection of infected cancer cells. Since sporadic tumors are unlikely to express viral antigens, observed immune responses in such models rather reflect surveillance of virus-induced cancer which has been already shown to exist (Klein and Klein, 1977).

Although extensive research has been carried out on studying the interaction between tumors and the immune system, no mouse model exists allowing the adjustable induction of an oncogene *in vivo* at a distinct time point and with restricted expression to a defined location in the body in the absence of acute inflammation. Such a model would simulate sporadic tumor development as it occurs in humans more accurately and thus, enables the proof of concept of cancer immune surveillance.

1.7   Tumorigenesis by SV40 large T and its application in animal models

Tumor development is a multi-step process that is often based on a defective cell cycle control leading to uncontrolled cell proliferation. During that time, additional mutations are acquired that facilitate the transformation of pre-malignant cells into malignant cells (e.g. Lengauer et al., 1998).

Eddy et al. discovered in the 1960s an oncogenic substance in the extract of kidney cells from a rhesus monkey (*Macaca mulatta*) that induced tumor formation upon injection into newborn hamsters (Eddy et al., 1962). The oncogenic substance in this extract was identified as simian virus 40 (SV40), a polyoma virus whose genome encodes, next to structural and regulatory proteins, three tumor antigens: the small T (174 amino acids, aa), the large T (708 aa) and the 17K T antigen. All three proteins are expressed from a common precursor mRNA which is differentially spliced and results in expression of proteins that share the amino-terminal domain, including the first 82 aa, but contain different carboxy-terminal regions (Saenz-Robles et al., 2001). Albeit, only large T (Tag) is sufficient to induce cellular transformation, whereas small T has accessory functions and did not induce transformation in cell culture assays when it was expressed alone (Bikel et al., 1987; Stewart and Bacchetti, 1991). Intriguingly, even a truncated form of Tag containing aa 1 to 137 is sufficient to induce carcinoma in transgenic mice (Tevethia et al., 1997).

Tag-mediated cellular transformation is attributed to three domains of Tag: a C-terminal region binding to p53 (Lane and Crawford, 1979; Linzer and Levine, 1979), a retinoblastoma protein-binding region (DeCaprio et al., 1988) and a J region recruiting and activating the cellular chaperon hsc70 (Brodsky and Pipas, 1998) (Fig. 1.2a). The proteins p53 and retinoblastoma protein (Rb), are tumor suppressors that play central roles in cell cycle regulation. Binding of Tag to the tumor suppressor p53 leads to accumulation of p53 in the nucleus, reflecting a p53-mediated, DNA damage-induced cell cycle arrest (Tanaka et al., 2000). p53 acts as transcription factor inducing expression of effector genes, which are either negative regulators of cell cycle progression, e.g. p21, or apoptosis-promoting genes, e.g. BAX and BAC (Vogelstein et al., 2000). Increased levels of p53 leads to increased expression of p21

(Nakanishi et al., 2000) which acts as universal cyclin kinase inhibitor and hinders the entry into S-phase of cell cycle by binding to cyclin/CDK complexes (Xiong et al., 1993). Maintenance of the cell cycle arrest is observed until repair of the DNA damage (Kastan et al., 1991). If the DNA damage is irreparable, p53 induces programmed cell death in the affected cells (Yonish-Rouach et al., 1991). However, inhibition of p53 through binding of Tag blocks stress-induced apoptosis and cell cycle arrest triggered e.g. by abnormal Rb inhibition or DNA damage (Ahuja et al., 2005).

Rb protein family members, Rb, p107 and p130, have growth-suppressive functions mediated by binding to the eukaryotic transcription factor E2F family members (E2Fs). Binding of Rb results in functional inactivation of E2Fs and inhibits entry of cells into and progression through the cell cycle. However, if Tag binds to Rb protein family members, this complex dissociates and E2Fs are released, which permit expression of E2F-regulated genes and cell cycle progression (DeCaprio et al., 1988). Additionally, Rb proteins are released from E2Fs through phosphorylation by cyclin-dependent kinases (CDKs).

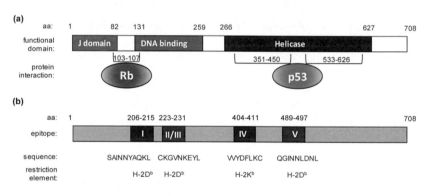

Figure 1.2 SV 40 large T antigen
(a) SV40 large T (Tag) consists of different functional domains whereby its transforming capacity is mainly mediated by interaction with the cellular tumor suppressor proteins p53 and Rb. Amino acid (aa) sequences for functional and binding domains are indicated. Figure partially adapted from (DeCaprio and Garcea, 2013). (b) Tag harbors 5 described H-2^b-restricted epitopes. The immunodominant epitope IV is restricted to H-2K^b whereas the subdominant epitopes I and II/III and the immunorecessive epitope V are restricted to H-2D^b. Figure modified from (Mylin et al., 2000).

The discovery of SV40 large T and its underlying transforming capacity gave scientists a powerful tool to investigate cancer in a mouse model, not only in *in vitro* cell culture experiments. In contrast to other mouse cancer models, only a single transgene is required for tumorigenesis, and thus make SV40 models faster and cost effective to produce. In 1974, Jaenisch and Mintz produced the first transgenic mouse model by microinjection of SV40 viral DNA into mouse blastocysts (Jaenisch and Mintz, 1974). Although tumor formation was not observed, SV40 viral DNA was detected in tissues of adult mice. 10 years later, the first transgenic mouse model that resulted in primary tumor formation was published by

Brinster et al. After microinjection of a plasmid containing SV40 early region genes and a metallothionein fusion gene, all mice developed tumors within the choroid plexus in the brain (Brinster et al., 1984). Since then SV40 large T has been expressed in different organs in a variety of transgenic mice, including pancreas (Hanahan, 1985), liver (Dubois et al., 1991), prostate (Greenberg et al., 1995), lung (Magdaleno et al., 1997) and ovary (Connolly et al., 2003).

A further great advantage is that SV40 large T mouse models of cancer allow the study of T cell responses *in vivo*. The immunogenic potential of Tag was analyzed in C57BL/6 mice by Mylin et al. and revealed four $H2^b$-restricted epitopes (Fig. 1.2b). *In vivo* Tag-specific responses are dominated by epitope IV-specific $CD8^+$ T cells ($H-2K^b$-restricted), followed by $CD8^+$ T cell responses against the subdominant epitopes I and II/III (both $H-2D^b$-restricted). Another $H-2D^b$-restricted epitope V elicited only a $CD8^+$ T cell response *in vivo* when the other immunodominant epitopes were absent, and thus, it is a recessive epitope (Mylin et al., 1995; Mylin et al., 2000). In summary, the proposed hierarchy is as followed: epitope IV (residues 404-411) > epitope I (residues 206-2015) > epitope II/III (residues 223-231) > epitope V (residues 489-497). Recently, $CD4^+$ T cell epitopes that give rise to an immune response in C57BL/6 mice, were identified by Christian Schön of the Blankenstein group (data unpublished).

The ability of SV40 to cause cancer in humans remains controversial. It is proposed that SV40 infections established in humans primarily because of exposure to contaminated oral polio vaccines (Carbone et al., 2003). However, detection of SV40 DNA and protein in human cancers, e.g. malignant mesothelioma and brain tumors, does not necessarily link viral infection to tumorigenesis. This is supported by the finding that neither tumor incidence in individuals that received contaminated vaccines is increased nor that SV40 infections are widespread in the population and have a direct role in human cancer (Institute of Medicine Immunization Safety Review, 2002).

1.8 Gene regulation by the Tet system

Transgenic mouse models that facilitate a spatiotemporal gene expression are a powerful approach to understand and explore the biological function of specific genes during development and tumorigenesis. The most extensively applied systems for controlled gene expression in mammalian cells are the Cre/*lox* P system and the tetracycline (Tet) system. In contrast to the Cre-mediated induction of gene expression, which is irreversible, gene expression by the Tet-system is reversible and permits a time-restricted and quantitative adjustable manner. Thus, Tet-regulated, temporal gene expression is a useful tool in cancer research, e.g. in testing the addiction of tumors to oncogenes or their evolved oncogene-independence at later stages of tumor progression (Jonkers and Berns, 2004).

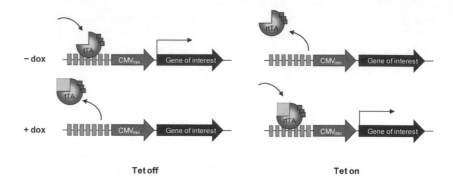

Tet off   **Tet on**

Figure 1.3 Gene regulation by the Tet on/Tet off system
The Tet off and Tet on transactivators (tTA/rtTA) consist of the Tet repressor binding domain (*tetR*, green) derived from *E. coli* fused to three consecutive minimal transcription activation domains derived from Herpes simplex virus (HSV) protein VP16 (blue boxes). For transcription of the gene of interest, the tTA and the rtTA, respectively, must bind to their cognate promoter, a heptamerized Tet operator (*tetO*) sequence (light grey boxes) which is joint to a minimal CMV promoter. The tTA is active in the absence of dox (yellow square) and binds to the promoter but dissociates from it in the presence of dox (left panel). In contrast, the rtTA exhibits opposite properties due to five point mutations and facilitates transcription in the presence of dox (right panel).

Gossen and Bujard developed the Tet-system that is based on regulatory elements of the Tn*10* tetracycline-resistant operon (*tetO*) of *E. coli* (Gossen and Bujard, 1992). The *tet* repressor is fused to the activating domain of virion protein 16 of herpes simplex virus (VP16) and thus, a tet-controlled transcription activator (tTA) is formed which can be constitutively expressed under the control of a cell- or tissue-specific promoter of interest. For tTA-driven expression, the target gene must be linked to the minimal promoter sequence of the human cytomegalovirus (CMV) combined with heptamerized *tetO* sequences. This 'Tet-off' system permits gene expression in the absence of tetracycline or it derivates, e.g. doxycycline (dox), by binding of the tTA to the *tetO* elements and subsequent transcription initiation through the active CMV promoter. By contrast, presence of dox induces conformational changes of the tTA that leads to its dissociation from *tetO* and termination of target gene transcription (Fig. 1.3, left). Because target gene expression in the 'Tet-off' system is dependent on dox administration, it is not ideally suited when the target gene needs to be kept silent during embryonic and neonatal stages until adult-onset. Long-term dox application might have undesired effects and additionally, the time of target gene expression depends on the clearance of dox from the system that may take several days. To compensate for those limitations, Gossen and Bujard developed a 'Tet-on' system, in which a reverse tTA (rtTA) that harbors a mutant *tet* repressor is constitutively silent. Activation of target gene transcription requires the presence of dox, that induces conformational changes and subsequent *tetO*-binding of the rtTA (Fig. 1.3, right). However, the rtTA exhibited initial limitations, most notably insufficient inducibility in some organs, instability and residual *tetO*-binding in the absence of dox, which led to elevated background promoter activity. A novel rtTA mutant (rtTA2^S-M2) showed reduced basal activity and a ten-fold increased dox sensitivity and eliminated the previous limitations (Urlinger et al., 2000).

1.9 Non-invasive bioluminescent imaging

Bioluminescence imaging (BLI) is a technology that has been developed in the past decades as a powerful tool for molecular imaging of small laboratory animals. It enables study of ongoing biological processes *in vivo* in a spatial and temporal manner. The technique is based on detection of visible light emission in living organisms. Due to the oxidation of a molecular substrate by the enzyme luciferase, light is emitted which can then be quantified by a high-sensitive cooled charge-coupled device (CCD) (Rice et al., 2001). Sensitivity of light detection depends on several factors, including level of luciferase expression and distance of labelled cells in the tissue from detection device (Wilson and Hastings, 1998). There is an approximate 10-fold loss of photon intensity per centimeter of tissue depth. However, Edinger et al. reported that as few as 100 to 1000 luciferase labelled cells injected into peritoneal cavity of white mice can be detected by BLI (Edinger et al., 1999). According to this sensitive measure, BL imaging facilitates detection of small malignant lesions before they become palpable and provides a great advantage in long-term monitoring of transplanted tumor cells and tumor growth *in vivo*.

Sensitivity of BL imaging is greatly influenced by the properties of emitted light and selection of a luciferase with light of ideal wavelength is important. The luciferase from the North American firefly (*Photinus pyralis*) is the most commonly used reporter gene applied for BL imaging approaches. Cloned in 1985 by de Wet et al. (de Wet et al., 1985), the light produced by this firefly luciferase has a peak at wavelength of 620 nm. Thus, it shows optimal properties for tissue penetration, since only light with wavelengths above 600 nm is not absorbed by hemoglobin in the tissue. In contrast to fluorescent reporters, bioluminescent reporter systems, e.g. firefly luciferase, exhibit a minimal background signal from animal tissue and even weak signals with a high signal-to-background ratio can be detected (Troy et al., 2004). The combination of relatively high sensitivity with minimal background signals and the non-invasiveness of BL imaging enables real-time *in vivo* monitoring of tumor cell growth at a stage reflecting neoplastic lesions. In consequence, the effect of the immune system on growing tumor cells can be studied in a spatiotemporal manner. Further, BL imaging allows quantitative and sensitive evaluation of tumor regression upon new therapeutic strategies in preclinical animal models.

The application of dual-reporter systems consisting of different luciferases that convert specific substrates and produce light with variant wavelengths, enabled monitoring of different cell populations simultaneously in one individual animal (Mezzanotte et al., 2011). Another example is the transgenic dual-luciferase reporter mouse which allows longitudinal and functional monitoring of T cells *in vivo*. By expression of a constitutive luciferase and a NFAT (nuclear factor of activated T cells)-dependent luciferase, migration and activation of T cells can be visualized (Szyska et al., 2018).

2 Aims

To date, only inadequate models are available for the proof of the cancer immune surveillance hypothesis and for answering the question at which time point during sporadic tumor formation the immune system interacts with emerging cancer cells. Several studies using experimental mouse models suggest a T cell-mediated immune surveillance, but they exhibited distinct limitations: the tumor antigens remained elusive, the T cell responses were not analyzed in the primary host, experiment-intrinsic artifacts interfered with occurring immune responses and/or long tumor latency counteracted the analysis of T cell responses during early tumorigenesis. Therefore, a model would be desirable which enables the study of T cell responses against a neoantigen expressed by only few cancer cells under non-inflammatory conditions. Such a model would simulate sporadic tumor formation as it occurs in humans.

1. **Establishment of a mouse cancer transplantation model enabling the analysis of immune responses in the absence of acute inflammation**

The first part of the presented work describes the generation and characterization of a novel transplantation model in which oncogene/antigen expression is adjustable *in vivo*. Besides the phenotypic characterization of the applied cancer cell lines, intensive studies were performed to exclude any unintended tumor antigen expression which would provoke a T cell response due to the inoculation-induced inflammation. Based on the established transplantation model, all further analyses were conducted.

2. **Study of CD8$^+$ T cell responses against a neoantigen expressed in the absence of acute inflammation: Is there immunity or tolerance?**

The second part of the presented work addresses the question whether there is immune surveillance against neoantigens which are expressed by cancer cells in the absence of acute inflammation. By application of the proposed transplantation model, antigen-specific CD8$^+$ T cell responses were followed in immunocompetent hosts and the kinetics of tumor progression and rejection were analyzed by non-invasive bioluminescent imaging.

3. **Underlying mechanisms leading to priming and induction of neoantigen-specific CD8$^+$ T cells expressed in the absence of acute inflammation**

It is on debate whether direct priming of CD8$^+$ T cells by cancer cells results in an efficient cytotoxic T cell response. Therefore, the third part of the presented work investigates potential mechanisms of T cell priming that play a role in induction of neoantigen-specific T cell responses in the absence of acute inflammation.

3 Results

3.1 Selection and characterization of transplantable cancer cell lines allowing *in vivo* studies of T cell responses against a neoantigen

3.1.1 Establishment of cancer cell lines with conditional oncogene/antigen expression

This study aimed to select cancer cell lines suitable for a transplantation model allowing the study of tumor antigen-specific T cell responses against a neoantigen under resting conditions. Addressing this question, it was of great importance that the cell line of interest possesses a conditionally expressed tumor-specific antigen and cancer cell proliferation can be tightly regulated. Furthermore, the tumor specific antigen should harbor epitopes that can induce functional T cell responses in mice.

For this purpose, cancer cell line TC200.09 was used (Anders et al., 2011). TC200.09 cancer cells express SV40 large T antigen (Tag) which is fused to the reporter gene firefly luciferase (Luc) by a peptide linker, consisting of glycine-serine (G_4S_3) repeats (TagLuc). Expression of TagLuc fusion protein in TC200.09 cancer cells is controlled by a tetracycline responsive element (TRE) in the promoter region and depends on the presence of an active transactivator (rtTA) (Urlinger et al., 2000). Further, a loxP site-flanked stop cassette separates the promoter and TagLuc to prevent transcription and expression of TagLuc in the absence of tetracyclines, such as dox (Fig. 3.1A). Suitability of the TC200.09 cancer cell line for the proposed transplantation model was perceived by an *in vitro* observation: Although the cancer-driving antigen TagLuc was inactivated by dox withdrawal, a fraction of cancer cells did not undergo apoptosis and survived. Moreover, TagLuc expression was re-inducible by dox administration, and cells proliferated again (Figure 3.1B).

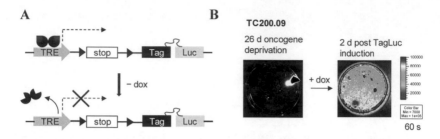

Figure 3.1 Regulation of TagLuc expression and proliferation in TC200.09 cancer cells by dox and re-inducibility of TagLuc expression after dox deprivation
(A) Proliferation of TC200.09 cancer cells depends on the expression of the cancer-driving oncogene TagLuc. TagLuc is expressed after binding of the dox-activated transactivator rtTA (black dimer) to elements of the TRE promoter (grey box), which results in transcription of TagLuc. Abrogation of rtTA binding is induced by dox withdrawal and results in stop of TagLuc transcription. Prevention of TagLuc transcription by the stop cassette (white box) may not be complete due to spontaneous deletions in single transgene copies. (B) TC200.09 cancer cells survived oncogene inactivation and after 4 weeks of oncogene deprivation, TagLuc was re-expressed in resting cancer cells. 5×10^6 cells were cultured in a 10 cm dish for 26 days (d) in the absence of dox. TagLuc was induced by administration of dox (1 μg/ml). TagLuc signal was measured by BL imaging (exposure time: 60 s) and is shown for 1 of 2 culture plates at the indicated time point.

Since this project aimed to study only T cell responses related to Tag, which is regulated by dox, potential T cell epitopes that cannot be regulated in the described model, were removed. The stop cassette chloramphenicol acetyltransferase (CAT), which is expressed in TC200.09 cancer cells, can harbor such T cell epitopes. Therefore, excision of CAT was performed by transient gene transfer in cultured cells with a Cre recombinase-encoding adenovirus (Ad-Cre) (Fig. 3.2A). Subsequently, single cell clones were generated and tested for stop cassette excision by polymerase chain reaction (PCR) using recombination-specific primers (Fig. 3.2B). From the tested clones, TC200.09-AdCre clone 4F5, referred to as 'clone 4', exhibited deletion of CAT and was chosen for further analysis and experiments.

In addition to cancer cell line clone 4, a second cell line was selected that displayed the same feature of survival upon temporary oncogene inactivation *in vitro*. Cancer cell line TTC #3055 was isolated from a sporadic tumor occurring 435 days (d) after dox treatment in a triple-transgenic mouse (TRE[loxP]stop[loxP]TagLuc xCAG-rtTA xTyrCre). Importantly, TTC #3055 cancer cells do not express tyrosinase anymore. Consequently, Cre recombinase is also not expressed by those cells (Anders et al., 2017). Different from clone 4 cancer cells, recombination-specific PCR revealed a partial deletion of the stop cassette (Fig. 3.2C). Due to different copy numbers, the stop cassette might be deleted in some, but not in all copies of the transgene. Further, TTC #3055 cancer cells were not cloned after tumor isolation and thus, it is a heterogeneous cell line that likely comprises cancer cells with and without stop cassette deletion.

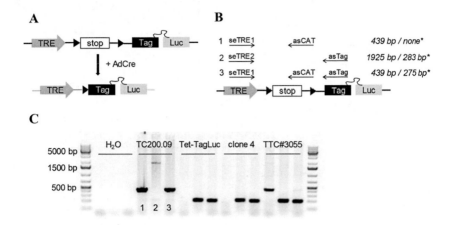

Figure 3.2 Generation of a cancer cell line that survives temporary TagLuc inactivation
(A) Schematic overview of clone 4 generation. A loxP site –flanked stop cassette that separates the TRE from TagLuc, was excised by application of AdCre, and subsequent single cell cloning was performed. (B) Set of primers used to detect recombination of stop cassette by PCR. seTRE1 and seTRE2 primers bind to the TRE promoter region of the transgene, asCAT primer binds within the stop cassette, and asTag primer binds to Tag sequence. Size of PCR products are depicted for each primer combination. Products marked with an asterisk (*) are only amplified after stop cassette deletion. as, antisense, se, sense. (C) PCR to test cell lines for stop cassette deletion reveals complete deletion in clone 4 cancer cells, but only partial deletion in TTC #3055 cancer cells. Controls: TC200.09 (negative control), Tet-TagLuc (positive control, deleted stop cassette). Depicted numbers indicate the primer pairs shown in (B), which were used for detection of stop cassette deletion.

3.1.2 Conditional oncogene inactivation resulted in decreased TagLuc expression and proliferative arrest of cancer cells

Sustained oncogene expression is often required for tumor maintenance, a phenomenon known as oncogene addiction (Weinstein and Joe, 2008). According to this, it has not yet been tested whether TagLuc expression in clone 4 and TTC #3055 cancer cells is essential for survival *in vitro*. In both cancer cell lines, TagLuc expression depend on the presence of the transactivator rtTA, which is activated only in the presence of dox. Dox induces conformational changes of the transactivator, that subsequently binds to the promoter and induces transcription of TagLuc (Fig. 3.3A). The effect of TagLuc inactivation by dox withdrawal was studied in both cancer cell lines. Dox deprivation affected proliferation of both cancer cell lines and resulted in reduced living cells over time (Fig. 3.3B). Counting living cells before and after 14 d of dox deprivation revealed that ≈ 23 % of clone 4 cancer cells survived temporary TagLuc inactivation *in vitro* (Fig. 3.3C).

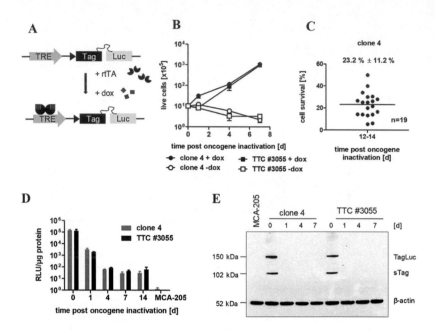

Figure 3.3 Decreased TagLuc expression and proliferation upon dox withdrawal in cancer cells
(A) Clone 4 and TTC #3055 cancer cells express a TagLuc fusion protein under control of a tetracycline-sensitive promoter. Expression of the cancer-driving antigen is dependent on a dox-inducible, active transactivator binding to the TRE element of the promoter. (B) Effect of dox withdrawal on proliferation of cancer cells was examined by live cell count. 1×10^6 cells were seeded in cell culture flasks (duplicates) and live cells were counted at indicated days post oncogene inactivation. (C) Quantification of viable clone 4 cancer cells 12 to 14 days (d) post oncogene inactivation was performed by trypan blue staining. Percentage of surviving clone 4 cells was calculated in relation to initial cell number before oncogene inactivation. Results from 19 independent experiments are displayed. (D) Cancer cells were grown in the presence (d0) or absence (d1-d14) of dox. 1×10^6 cells (duplicates) were analyzed for luciferase activity upon oncogene inactivation. Cells were harvested, protein concentration was determined, and luciferase activity was measured in a luminometer (exposure time: 1 s). Results from 3 independent experiments are displayed as relative light units (RLU; ± SD). MCA-205: negative control. (E) TagLuc protein expression in clone 4 and TTC #3055 cancer cells cultured in the presence or absence of dox was detected by Western blot. Proteins were isolated from cells at d 0 to d 7 post TagLuc inactivation and loaded on a SDS gel. Antibodies to detect proteins on nitrocellulose membrane: monoclonal mouse anti-SV40 T antigen antibody and rabbit anti-ß-actin antibody. MCA-205 served as negative control (exposure time: 1 min).

Inactivation of TagLuc expression by dox deprivation expectedly led to a decreased luciferase activity in clone 4 and TTC #3055 cancer cells (Fig. 3.3D). Compared to the TagLuc negative cell line MCA-205, a low, residual luciferase activity was still detectable in both cancer cell lines. However, luciferase activity after 14 d of dox withdrawal was more than three logs lower compared to cancer cells cultured in the presence of dox. In contrast, already one day post oncogene inactivation, Tag protein expression was not detectable in Western Blot analysis (Fig. 3.3E). After incubation with monoclonal anti-SV40 T antigen antibody, an additional band with a molecular size of ≈ 100 kDa was detected on the membrane. Considering the molecular weight of firefly luciferase (62 kDa) and Tag (94 kDa), it is suggested that the antibody bound a splicing product of TagLuc that is likely to be Tag (termed 'sTag').

In order to investigate the proliferative arrest induced by withdrawal of the cancer-driving oncogene TagLuc through dox deprivation, a 5-bromo-2'-deoxyuridine (BrdU) incorporation assay was performed. After 7 d of TagLuc inactivation, more than 70 % of cancer cells that survived dox deprivation arrested in the G1 phase of cell cycle. For comparison, 50 % of cancer cells 'on dox' were detected in the G1 phase. Moreover, whereas ≈ 40 % of cancer cells 'on dox' were detected in the S phase of cell cycle, only up to 0.5 % of cancer cells were detected in S phase at 7 d post TagLuc inactivation confirming the observed proliferative arrest (Fig. 3.4A-D).

Next, the observed cell cycle arrest was investigated further. Macroscopic analysis of clone 4 or TTC #3055 cancer cells upon TagLuc inactivation by light microscopy revealed a partial change of cellular morphology starting at d 3 post TagLuc inactivation. Cells became enlarged, flattened and irregular in shape, which is characteristic for senescent cells (Kuilman et al., 2010) (Fig. 3.5A, TTC #3055 cancer cells: see Appendix). Analysis of senescence-associated (SA) proteins by Western blot showed a diverse expression pattern of common senescence markers. Both cancer cell lines exhibited an increased expression of histone 3 trimethylated K9 (H3K9me) at d 1 post TagLuc inactivation (Fig. 3.5B), which is described for senescent cells. In contrast to this, p21, whose expression is usually down-regulated in senescent cells, was only expressed at low amounts in both cancer cell lines 'on dox' and remarkably stronger expressed in TagLuc-inactivated TTC #3055 cancer cells. Further, two bands at d 0 and d 1 post TagLuc induction were detected after incubation with monoclonal anti-p21 antibodies. It is suggested that those two bands represented a hypo- and a hyper-phosphorylated form of p21 (Dash and El-Deiry, 2005). Another SA marker, p16, whose expression is usually up-regulated in senescent cells, was down-regulated in both cancer cell lines upon TagLuc inactivation (Fig. 3.5C). Those results suggest a proliferative arrest displaying some but not all features of senescence.

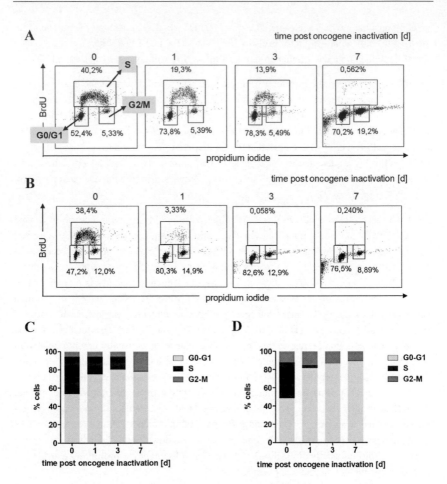

Figure 3.4 Surviving cancer cells arrested in G1 phase of cell cycle after TagLuc inactivation
(A, B) BrdU incorporation by clone 4 (A) or TTC #3055 (B) cancer cells upon oncogene inactivation was detected to identify number of cells in different cell cycle phases. Cancer cells were stained with propidium iodide (50 µg/ml) to distinguish single-stranded from double-stranded DNA, and with an APC-labelled. monoclonal anti-BrdU antibody to detect BrdU incorporation into DNA. After a 1-hour (h) pulse with BrdU (10 µM) cells were harvested, stained and analyzed by flow cytometry. Results shown are representative from 1 out of 3 experiments. Cells within different cell cycle phases are gated within black frames. Grey boxes in the first dot plot mark the cell cycle phases exemplarily. **(C, D)** Proportion of cells in different cell cycle phases upon oncogene inactivation was identified by BrdU incorporation. One representative out of 3 experiments is displayed for clone 4 cancer cells (C) and TTC #3055 cancer cells (D), respectively.

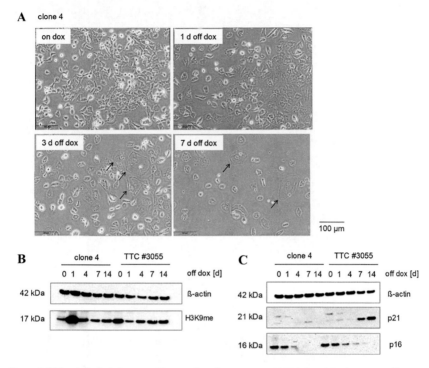

Figure 3.5 Morphological changes and expression of senescence-associated proteins in cancer cells upon TagLuc inactivation

(A) Morphological changes of clone 4 cancer cells upon TagLuc inactivation were detected by phase-contrast light microscopy (40x magnification). Black arrows indicate enlarged and flattened cells with irregular shape. (B, C) Senescence-associated (SA) protein expression in clone 4 and TTC #3055 cancer cells cultured in the presence or absence of dox was detected by Western blot. Proteins were isolated from cells at d 0 to d 14 post TagLuc inactivation and loaded on a SDS gel. Antibodies to detect proteins on nitrocellulose membrane: monoclonal mouse anti-SV40 T antigen antibody, polyclonal rabbit anti-p16, anti-p21 and anti-histone 3(tri methyl K9) (H3K9me) antibody, and rabbit anti-ß-actin antibody. (exposure time: 1 min). Results shown are representative for 1 of 3 independent experiment (p16, p21) and 1 of 2 independent experiments (H3K9me).

In summary, clone 4 and TTC #3055 cancer cells exhibited a unique property by surviving temporary inactivation of the cancer-driving oncogene TagLuc. The ability to revert the senescent-like proliferative arrest via dox-mediated TagLuc re-induction made them ideally suitable for the proposed transplantation model in which the cancer-driving oncogene/antigen TagLuc will be re-induced *in vivo* after a resting period of 3 to 4 weeks. In this setting, the oncogene/antigen is not expressed during the acute inflammation induced by cancer cell inoculation.

3.1.3 Cancer cells were not recognized by Tag-specific CD8$^+$ T cells *in vitro* upon oncogene/antigen inactivation

It was of great importance for the postulated model to prevent antigen expression by the cancer cells 'off dox' that may be recognized by T cells of immunocompetent hosts upon inoculation. Therefore, both cancer cell lines were tested for their potential to activate Tag peptide I (pI)-specific CD8$^+$ T cells *in vitro*. Clone 4 or TTC #3055 cancer cells were cultured for 14 d in the absence of dox. After 5 d of co-culture with CFSE-labelled TCR-I transgenic T cells, which recognize Tag epitope I, no antigen-specific T cell proliferation was detected. Control cancer cells cultured 'on dox' led to proliferation of CFSE-labelled TCR-I T cells, which was observed as dilution of CFSE fluorescence (Fig. 3.6A, FACS plots for TTC #3055 not shown).

Supernatants of the co-culture were analyzed in an IFN-γ ELISA (enzyme-linked immunosorbent assay) to test whether T cells in this assay produced IFN-γ upon activation. Consistent with the results of the CFSE dilution assay, T cells only produced IFN-γ if they were activated through TagLuc-expressing cancer cells. T cells co-cultured with cancer cells 'off dox' secreted negligible amounts of IFN-γ, which were comparable to the background secretion of IFN-γ by TCR-I T cells alone (Fig. 3.6B).

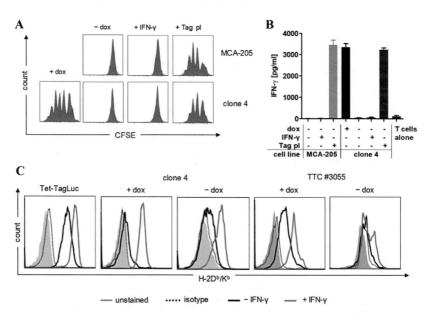

Figure 3.6 No recognition of TagLuc-inactivated clone 4 cancer cells by TCR-I T cells *in vitro*
(A) Clone 4 cancer cells were cultured for 7 d in the absence of dox or, as control, in the presence of dox. $1x10^5$ cancer cells were co-cultured with CFSE-labelled SV40-TCR-I transgenic splenocytes for 5 d (triplicates). To detect Tag-specific T cell proliferation, splenocytes were stained after 5 d of co-culture with monoclonal anti-CD3 and anti-CD8 antibodies, and CFSE dilution was measured by flow cytometry (gate: $CD3^+CD8^+$ lymphocytes). CFSE flourescence is displayed as histogram for an effector/target (E/T) cell ratio of 5:1. MCA-205 cancer cells served as a negative control. IFN-γ (100 ng/ml) was added to augment MHC class I molecule expression on cancer cells. Tag peptide I (10^{-6} M) was loaded on cancer cells as a positive control. (B) IFN-γ production by SV40-TCR-I transgenic T cells after 5 d co-culture with cancer cells (shown in Fig. 3.6A) was detected by ELISA. Results displayed are from a co-culture with an E/T ratio of 5:1 (triplicates). Shown is IFN-γ concentration [pg/ml] ± SEM. (C) MHC-class I molecule H-2K^b/H-2D^b expression on clone 4 and TTC #3055 cancer cells, either treated with INF-γ (24 h, 100 ng/ml) or left untreated, was detected by flow cytometry. Shown are representative histograms for each cell line from 1 of 2 independent experiments. Antibodies: 1st: biotin-mouse anti-H-2K^b/H-2D^b (1:100); 2nd: anti-streptavidin (1:100). Filled grey line: unstained, dotted line: isotype control, black line: - IFN-γ, blue line: + IFN-γ.

In addition, clone 4 and TTC #3055 cancer cells were tested for expresion ofMHC class I molecules and the ability to increase this expression upon IFN-γ stimulation. It was necessary to exclude that after 14 d of oncogene inactivation, antigens presented on the cancer cells were generally not recognized by T cells because of a diminished expression of MHC class I molecules on cancer cells 'off dox'. Although both cancer cell lines had a general low MHC class I molecule expression independent of TagLuc inactivation, its expression was up-regulated upon IFN-γ stimulation (Fig. 3.6C). However, when IFN-γ was added exogenously within the T cell antigen recognition assy, it did not lead to recognition of residual, low TagLuc expressed on cancer cells 'off dox' by TCR-I T cells (Fig. 3.6A).

In summary, these results indicate that eminently low TagLuc expression on cancer cells upon dox deprivation, as shown in Fig. 3.3D and detected only by a highly sensitive lucifer-ase activity assay, did not induce recognition by Tag-specific CD8$^+$ T cells. Furthermore, the displayed results show that even when IFN-γ upregulated the expression of MHC class I molecules on cancer cells, as it would occur during inoculation-induced acute inflammation, it did not result in unintended Tag-specific CD8$^+$ T cell recognition.

3.2   Induction of Tag-specific CD8$^+$ T cell responses upon *de novo* TagLuc expression in the absence of acute inflammation

In the first part of this work, two cancer cell lines that appeared to be suitable for a trans-plantation model mimicking the immune response to sporadic cancer were characterized and established. In the following part, these two cancer cell lines were applied *in vivo* to investi-gate T cell responses against *de novo*-expressed TagLuc under resting conditions and in the absence of acute inflammation.

3.2.1 Cancer cells survived in immunodeficient mice upon oncogene inactivation and tumors grew out after re-induced TagLuc expression

First, survival and the ability of both cancer cell lines to express TagLuc again when inoculated into immunodeficient mice, was tested. For this purpose, cancer cells were cultured for 14 d in the absence of dox. Then, 1×10^5 cells were inoculated subcutaneously (s.c.) into Rag$^{-/-}$ mice. For prevention of excessive cell death in form of anoikis (Frisch and Francis, 1994), cancer cells were inoculated together with Matrigel containing a mixture of different extracellular matrix proteins (Kleinman et al., 1986). After 4 weeks, dox was adminstered to the mice and TagLuc expression was analyzed by BL imaging (Fig. 3.7A). Cells of both cancer cell lines, clone 4 and TTC #3055, survived *in vivo* and TagLuc induction in remaining cancer cells led to an immediate BL signal detectable already 1 d post dox administration (Fig. 3.7B, E).

BL signals increased over time and furthermore, re-induced TagLuc expression resulted in tumor outgrowth. Tumor growth was remarkably slower compared to other transplantation models, e.g. models transplanting MCA-induced tumors (e.g. shown in Shankaran et al., 2001; Swann et al., 2008). Tumors reached a size of 500 mm^3 after approximately 70 d post TagLuc induction for clone 4 and > 80 d for TTC #3055, respectively (Fig. 3.7C, F). This corresponded to a clinical relevant and detectable tumor size (Schreiber et al., 2006; Klein, 2009).

Taken together, these results demonstrate that clone 4 and TTC #3055 cancer cells survived several weeks *in vivo* despite persistent oncogene deprivation. Moreover, TagLuc expression was re-inducible in resting cancer cells and resulted in subsequent tumor outgrowth in immunodeficient mice. Tumor growth kinetics were notably slower compared to those observed in other transplantation models using e.g MCA-induced sarcoma or B16 melanoma cells (Hill and Littlejohn, 1971). According to this, the transplantation model simulated early phases of sporadic tumorigenesis more accurately because the progression of cancer cells from a malignant lesion to an established tumor is rather slow. Since these experiments were conducted in immundodeficient mice, it was tested next whether oncogene-deprived cancer cells survive in immunocompetent mice, and what is the consequence of TagLuc induction in cancer cells under resting conditions in these mice.

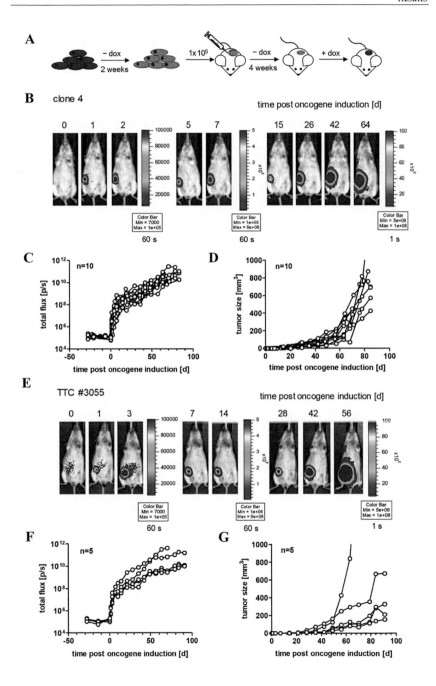

A

B clone 4

time post oncogene induction [d]

C n=10

D n=10

E TTC #3055

time post oncogene induction [d]

F n=5

G n=5

Figure 3.7 Induction of TagLuc in resting cancer cells led to tumor outgrowth in Rag$^{-/-}$ mice

(A) Scheme of mouse experiments is shown. Cancer cells are usually cultured for 14 d in the absence of dox to switch off TagLuc expression. If not indicated differently, 1×10^5 cancer cells in 10 mg/ml BD Matrigel^{TM} were inoculated s.c. into recipient mice and TagLuc was induced by dox administration after 4 weeks. (B) TagLuc expression in Rag$^{-/-}$ mice inoculated with oncogene-deprived clone 4 cancer cells after re-induction of TagLuc by dox adminstration (200 µg/ml) via drinking water. TagLuc signal was measured by BL imaging (exposure time: 1 s to 60 s) and followed over time. Pictures from one representative mouse are shown. (C) BL signal kinetic over time is displayed for each Rag$^{-/-}$ mouse inoculated with clone 4 cancer cells. Data shown from 3 independent experiments with total number of n=10 mice. (D) Tumor outgrowth in all Rag$^{-/-}$ mice is shown for clone 4 cancer cells. Tumor volume was measured with a caliper (formula: xyz/2). (E) TagLuc expression in Rag$^{-/-}$ mice inoculated with oncogene-deprived TTC #3055 cancer cells is shown. BL imaging pictures from one representative mouse are displayed. (F) BL signal kinetic over time is displayed for each Rag$^{-/-}$ mouse (n=5) inoculated with TTC #3055 cancer cells. Data from one experiment. (G) Tumor growth in Rag$^{-/-}$ mice shown in (F) is displayed.

3.2.2 TagLuc expression by resting cancer cells resulted in rapid BL signal induction followed by loss of BL signal in immunocompetent hosts

Testing the survival of cancer cells in immunocompetent hosts, clone 4 and TTC #3055 cancer cells were inoculated into CM2 mice. The use of CM2 mice as hosts was imperative because both cancer cell lines constitutively express the transactivator rtTA, which has been described as a rejection antigen in skin graft experiments by Anders et al. (Anders et al., 2011). Since CM2 mice express the transactivator rtTA as a transgene, T cells are tolerized to it and potential immune responses towards the cancer cells will not be caused by induction of rtTA-specific T cells. Based on the *in vitro* T cell antigen recognition assay (Fig. 3.6), it was hypothesized that inoculated cancer cells will not evoke an immune response in transactivator tolerant CM2 mice leading to rejection of the inoculated cancer cells. Therefore, both cancer cell lines were cultured *in vitro* for 14 d in the absence of dox in order to switch off TagLuc expression and cancer cells were subsequently inoculated into CM2 or Rag$^{-/-}$ mice. Mice were imaged weekly after inoculation to discover potential BL signals at the inoculation site. Such signals would indicate an unpreferred TagLuc expression before its experimental induction. No specific BL signals were detected at the inoculation site until 4 to 5 weeks post inoculation. In consequence, mice were administered dox via drinking water to induce TagLuc expression in resting cancer cells (= d 0). Already 1 d after TagLuc induction, an immediate BL signal was observed which increased over time (Fig. 3.8A, B). However, the BL signal started to decline between 10 and 14 d, and was finally lost in all immunocompetent CM2 mice until 21 d post TagLuc induction (Fig. 3.8). In contrast, BL signals in immunodeficient Rag$^{-/-}$ mice increased over time as it was already shown before (Fig. 3.7B, E).

In summary, survival of oncogene-deprived clone 4 or TTC #3055 cancer cells in CM2 mice was comparable to survival in Rag$^{-/-}$ mice, shown by a similar magnitude of the BL signal 1 d post TagLuc induction. In contrast to Rag$^{-/-}$ mice, that showed an increasing BL signal over time and final tumor outgrowth, BL signals in CM2 mice initially increased but declined within 2 weeks after TagLuc induction resulting in complete loss of BL signal. In the next section, it was examined whether Tag-specific CD8$^+$ T cells caused the observed BL signal loss and eradicated TagLuc-expressing cancer cells in CM2 mice.

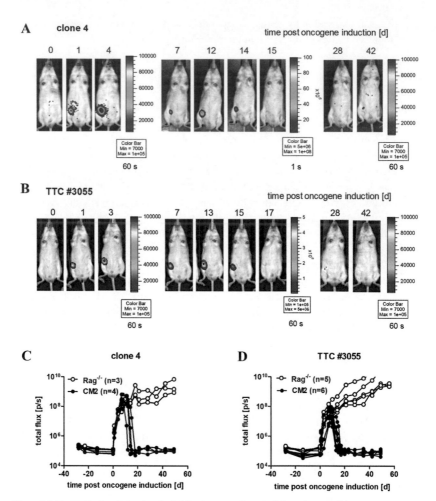

Figure 3.8 Rapid TagLuc induction in CM2 mice upon dox administration was followed by BL signal loss within 2 to 3 weeks

(A, B) TagLuc induction in CM2 mice 4 weeks after inoculation of clone 4 or TTC #3055 cancer cells is displayed. Cancer ells were cultured 14 d in the absence of dox and 1×10^5 cancer cells (in 10 mg/ml BD Matrigel[TM]) were injected s.c. TagLuc expression was measured over time (indicated in d post oncogene induction) by BL imaging (exposure time: 1 to 60 s) for individual mice. BL signal kinetic of one representative mouse inoculated with clone 4 cancer cells (A) or TTC #3055 cancer cells (B), respectively, is shown. **(C, D)** BL signal over time is displayed for each CM2 or $Rag^{-/-}$ (control) mouse inoculated with clone 4 cancer cells (C) or TTC #3055 cancer cells (D). Number of mice per group is indicated in the respective figures. Results for clone 4 cancer cells are representative from one out of 4 independent experiments with n=14 CM2 mice. Results for TTC #3055 cancer cells are obtained from one experiment.

3.2.3   BL signal loss in immunocompetent mice was accompanied by induction of Tag-specific CD8$^+$ T cells

The main issue of this work was to investigate whether the *de novo* expressed tumor-specific antigen TagLuc can induce a destructive T cell response in immunocompetent mice under resting conditions of the developing tumor. The cancer-driving oncogene/antigen Tag harbors five H-2^b-restricted CD8$^+$ T cell epitopes, whereby Tag-specific CD8$^+$ T cells recognizing the dominant epitope IV, restricted to H-2K^b, and the subdominant epitope I, restricted to H-2D^b, are found most abundantly (Mylin et al., 2000). The use of specific peptide/MHC class I (p/MHC) tetramers for these epitopes allowed to analyze CD8$^+$ T cells from peripheral blood of CM2 mice during the time of BL signal loss. It was assumed that the BL signal loss indicated a T cell-mediated cancer cell rejection. Addressing this, blood samples were stained 7−9 d, 10−12 d and 13−16 d post TagLuc induction. A distinct population of Tag pI- and pIV-specific CD8$^+$ T cells was detected in all CM2 mice inoculated with clone 4 (Fig. 3.9A) or TTC #3055 (Fig. 3.9B) cancer cells, respectively. The Tag pI or pIV/MHC tetramer$^+$ populations emerged approximately 10 d post TagLuc induction. Only in one mouse of each group, either inoculated with clone 4 or TTC #3055 cancer cells, Tag pI-specific CD8$^+$ T cells were detected already 7 d post TagLuc induction (Fig. 3.9C, D). The maximum percentage of Tag-specific CD8$^+$ T cells in individual mice varied between 0.2 % and 4 % for both CD8$^+$ T cell populations and was independent of the inoculated cancer cell line (Fig. 3.9C, D). Tag-specific CD8$^+$ T cell cells in peripheral blood of CM2 mice were not detected at d 0 and before TagLuc was induced (shown for mice inoculated with clone 4 cancer cells) suggesting a *de novo* induction of CD8$^+$ T cells observed at later time points.

Frequencies of Tag pI- and Tag pIV-specific CD8$^+$ T cells in CM2 mice were not according to the hierarchy described by Mylin et al. (Mylin et al., 2000). Displaying an inverse hierarchy, Tag pI-specific CD8$^+$ T cells were detected with overall slightly higher frequencies than Tag pIV-specific CD8$^+$ T cells.

The results presented in this chapter demonstrate that expression of the tumor-specific antigen TagLuc in the absence of acute inflammation induced a CD8$^+$ T cell response in immunocompetent hosts with a normal T cell repertoire. Moreover, the data show that those newly induced CD8$^+$ T cells comprised specificities against two different epitopes of Tag and led to rejection of TagLuc-expressing cancer cells.

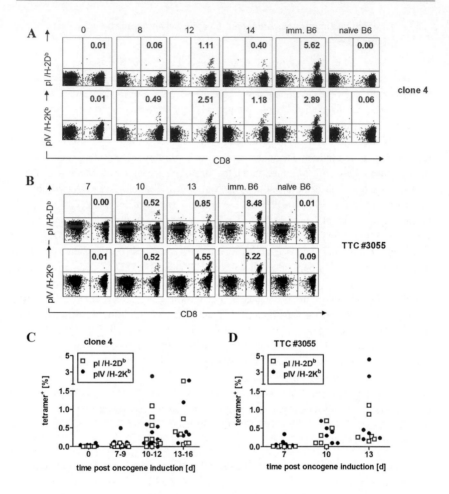

Figure 3.9 Induction of Tag-specific CD8[+] T cells in CM2 mice upon TagLuc re-expression on cancer cells

(A, B) Blood samples of CM2 mice previously inoculated with clone 4 cancer cells (A) or TTC #3055 cancer cells (B) were stained for Tag-specific T cells with H-2D^b tetramer loaded with Tag peptide I (pI/H-2D^b) or H-2K^b tetramer loaded with Tag peptide IV (pIV/H-2K^b). Staining of peripheral blood was performed at indicated days post TagLuc induction. Analysis was performed by flow cytometry. Gate: CD3[+] lymphocytes. Percentage of tetramer[+] cells out of CD8[+] lymphocyte population is indicated for each plot. Peripheral blood was additionally stained with mouse anti-CD3 and anti-CD8 antibodies. Negative control: C57BL/6 mouse ('naïve B6'), positive control: C57BL/6 mouse immunized with 5x10^6 Tet-TagLuc cancer cells i.p. ('imm. B6'). **(C, D)** Kinetic of Tag pI- and Tag pIV-specific T cell population detected by tetramer staining of peripheral blood cells from CM2 mice inoculated with clone 4 cancer cells (C) or TTC #3055 cancer cells (D) is shown. Results from staining performed at indicated time point post oncogene induction. Each symbol represents one individual mouse (clone 4: n=10, TTC #3055: n=6). Open squares: Tag pI/H-2D^b, black filled circles Tag pIV/H-2K^b.

3.2.4 TagLuc was induced *in vivo* only in a fraction of originally inoculated cancer cells

The transplantation model aimed to reflect sporadic cancer development in humans. One important issue was to induce expression of tumor-specific antigens already at early phases of tumorigenesis and hence, within a small cell population. Therefore, it was of large interest to explore the number of oncogene-deprived, resting cancer cells that survived 4 weeks of oncogene deprivation *in vivo*. Therefore, the number of clone 4 or TTC #3055 cancer cells 'on dox' that can still be detected by BL imaging was titrated *in vivo*. Albino C57BL/6 (B6) mice were inoculated with 1×10^2 to 1×10^5 cancer cells 'on dox' in Matrigel and BL signals were measured directly after inoculation. A quantifiable signal was detected starting from 1×10^3 inoculated cancer cells and increased in a linear manner up to 1×10^5 inoculated cancer cells for both cell lines (Fig. 3.10).

BL signals measured in Rag$^{-/-}$ and CM2 mice 1 d post TagLuc induction (Fig. 3.7 and Fig. 3.8) were mostly within the linear range that was measured in Fig. 3.10. This already implied that not all of the 1×10^5 inoculated cancer cells survived 4 weeks of oncogene deprivation caused by dox withdrawal *in vivo*. The equation of linear regression for each titrated cancer cell line was determined for a more precise quantification (depicted in diagrams of Fig. 3.10C, D). In this way, the number of cancer cells detected at d 1 post TagLuc induction in experiments shown beforehand (Fig. 3.7 and Fig. 3.8) was calculated. Since it is already known that cancer cell inoculation is accompanied by massive cell death (Schreiber et al., 2006), it was an expected finding that only a fraction of cells, both clone 4 and TTC #3055 cancer cells, were survived 4 weeks of oncogene deprivation after inoculation (Fig. 3.11A, B). Only minimal, non-significant differences in the number of surviving cancer cells were detected between Rag$^{-/-}$ and CM2 mice indicating no impact of the immune status on cancer cell survival. In general, TagLuc was induced in approximately 10 % of cancer cells compared to the number of cells which were inoculated 4 weeks before (Fig. 3.11C, D). Only one Rag$^{-/-}$ mouse inoculated with clone 4 cancer cells showed a BL signal corresponding closely to 1×10^5 cells (Fig. 3.11A). Cell numbers in which TagLuc was induced varied between $\approx 5 \times 10^3$ and $\approx 3 \times 10^4$ clone 4 cancer cells (Rag$^{-/-}$ outlier in group 'clone 4' was excluded) whereby TTC #3055 cancer cells showed slightly less numbers of surviving cells than clone 4 cancer cells (Fig. 3.11). The minor differences between both cancer cell lines might be caused by the different ability of transplanted cells to engraft *in vivo*. Clone 4 cancer cells originated from a cancer cell line that was passaged in a Rag$^{-/-}$ mouse to enhance *in vivo* tumor growth, whereas TTC #3055 cancer cells originated from a bulk culture of an isolated tumor that was never passaged *in vivo* for growth enhancement.

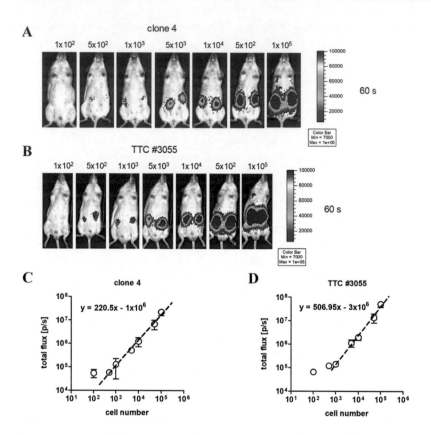

Figure 3.10 *In vivo* titration of clone 4 and TTC #3055 cancer cells 'on dox'
(A, B) Clone 4 cancer cells (A) or TTC #3055 cancer cells (B) (1×10^2 to 1×10^5, + 10 mg/ml BD Matrigel^{TM}) were inoculated s.c. into the left and right flank of albino B6 mice. BL signal of one representative mouse inoculated with the respective number of cells is shown for each cell line. (C, D) BL signals detected in albino B6 mice after inoculation with the respective number of cells for clone 4 cancer cells (C) and TTC #3055 cancer cells (D) is displayed. Results from 3 independent experiments are shown as mean total flux [p/s] (± SD). Equations depicted in graphs are derived from linear regression analysis. Dotted line is symbolic for the straight line based on the function and was inserted afterwards.

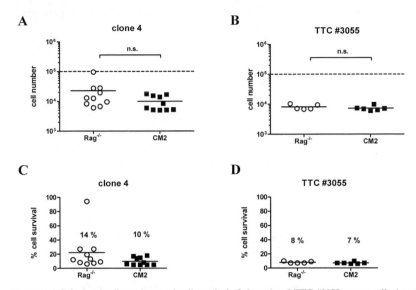

Figure 3.11 Calculated cell numbers and cell survival of clone 4 and TTC #3055 cancer cells 4 weeks after inoculation and TagLuc inactivation *in vivo*

(A, B) Number of clone 4 cancer cells (A) or TTC #3055 cancer cells (B) in which TagLuc was induced, was calculated. 1 d post oncogene induction, BL signal at inoculation site was meausred and calculated according to the BL signal from clone 4 or TTC #3055 cell titration in albino B6 mouse. The dashed line depicts the number of originally inoculated number of cells (= 1×10^5). Number of analyzed mice: clone 4: n=10 Rag$^{-/-}$, n=10 CM2; TTC #3055: n=5 Rag$^{-/-}$, n=6 CM2. Statistical analysis: unpaired t-test, significance: p-value $\leq$ 0.05. n.s.= not significant. **(C, D)** The percentage of surviving cells detected at d 1 post TagLuc induction was calculated for clone 4 cancer cells (C) and TTC #3055 cancer cells (D) and is displayed (+ mean). The outlier in Rag$^{-/-}$ group (clone 4) was excluded from calculation of mean % cell survival indicated in the diagram.

In summary, TagLuc was induced in a lower number of cells after 4 weeks of *in vivo* TagLuc inactivation compared to the number of originally inoculated cancer cells. In this context, it was argued that the presented transplantation model mimics a situation close to that found in sporadic tumors in which potentially immunogenic antigens are likely to be expressed in a small number of cells already at the beginning of tumorigenesis. The number of cells with re-induced TagLuc expression in the presented model presumably rather reflected a malignant lesion than an established tumor. In accordance with this, the significance of the model in recapitulating initial events of human sporadic cancer development was augmented.

3.2.5 TagLuc induction in a low number of cancer cells resulted in rejection and induction of Tag-specific CD8[+] T cells

Next, it was aimed to mimic a situation being close to that found in early phases of human sporadic cancer. Therefore, only 1×10^3 clone 4 cancer cells 'off dox' were inoculated into CM2 mice. According to the calculation of cancer cell survival in Fig. 3.10 and Fig. 3.11, it was assumed that TagLuc will be induced in only 10 % of inoculated cells which would correspond to 100 cancer cells. Thus, the proposed transplantation model would approach even closer a situation reflecting mutational events in early tumorigenesis. Another purpose of this experiment was to explore whether cancer cells can 'sneak through' T cell recognition if TagLuc is expressed by only few cancer cells, as it was described previously by Old et al. (Old et al., 1962).

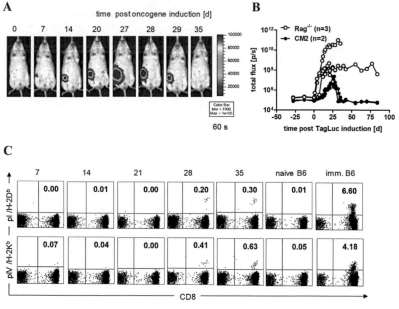

Figure 3.12 Recogntion and subsequent rejection of low numbers of TagLuc expressing cancer cells by Tag-specific CD8[+] T cells

(A) Low number of clone 4 cancer cells are rejected in CM2 mouse after TagLuc induction. 1×10^3 clone 4 cancer cells 'off dox' were inoculated s.c. and TagLuc expression was induced 4 weeks later. BL singal over time for one representative mouse is shown. **(B)** Individual BL signal kinetics of Rag$^{-/-}$ (n=3) and CM2 (n=2) are displayed. Results from one experiment are shown. **(C)** Detection of Tag-specific T cells in peripheral blood of CM2 mice by p/MHC tetramer staining. Blood was stained with anti-CD3 antibody, anti-CD8 antibody and p/MHC tetramers loaded with Tag pI or Tag pIV, at indicated time points post TagLuc induction.Shown are dot plots from on representative CM2 mouse. Frequencies of p/MHC tetramer$^+$ cells (of CD8$^+$) are indicated in %. Gate: CD3$^+$ lymphocytes. Results from one experiment with n=2 CM2 mice are shown. Negative control: naïve B6 mouse, positive control: B6 mouse immunized with 1×10^7 Tet-TagLuc cancer cells ('imm. B6').

Even though BL signals detected after TagLuc induction were initially lower in mice inoculated with 1×10^3 clone 4 cancer cells than in mice inoculated with 1×10^5 cells, TagLuc-expressing cancer cells were ultimately rejected (Fig. 3.12A, B). BL signals increased within ≈ 4 weeks post oncogene induction and then declined indicating cancer cell regression. It was tested whether the observed loss of BL signal correlated with induction of Tag-specific CD8$^+$ T cells, as it was shown for CM2 mice inoculated with 100-fold more cancer cells (Fig. 3.9). Staining of peripheral blood cells with Tag-specific p/MHC tetramers revealed an induction of Tag pI- and Tag pIV-specific CD8$^+$ T cells 35 d post TagLuc induction, but not at the time points analyzed before (Fig. 3.12C). Thus, the time point of appearance of Tag-specific CD8$^+$ T cells in peripheral blood was associated with the time point when TagLuc-expressing cancer cells were rejected.

Taken together, the data clearly indicate that TagLuc expression – even by very low numbers of cancer cells – induced Tag-specific CD8$^+$ T cells which rejected TagLuc$^+$ cancer cells under resting conditions. Further, the later onset of a destructive CD8$^+$ T cell response implied that a certain number of cancer cells that express enough TagLuc antigen, was required for priming of Tag-specific CD8$^+$ T cells.

3.2.6 Inoculation of TagLuc-inactivated cancer cells did not induce an unintended Tag-specific CD8$^+$ T cell response in CM2 mice

Using the transplantation model, it was aimed to study T cell responses against a *de novo* expressed tumor antigen in the absence of acute inflammation. Therefore, it was of outmost importance to exclude unintended antigen recognition by immune cells within the first weeks post cancer cell inoculation. It is well-described that cancer cell injection leads to massive coagulation necrosis and acute inflammation within the first 10 days (Schreiber et al., 2006). This was minimized by the use of Matrigel but could not be excluded completely in this study. In addition, antigen-specific T cells can be induced as well due to the inoculation-induced artifact influencing possible immune responses after TagLuc induction. Although T cell recognition of cancer cells 'off dox' *in vitro* was not observed (Fig. 3.6), it was tested whether minimal TagLuc expression in both cancer cells (Fig. 3.3D) is able to induce a Tag-specific CD8$^+$ T cell response before TagLuc induction *in vivo*. Clone 4 or TTC #3055 cancer cells were cultured for 12 d without dox to switch off TagLuc expression and were inoculated into CM2 mice. CFSE-labelled TCR-I transgenic splenocytes (1.9×10^6 CD8$^+$ Vβ7$^+$ cells per mouse) were transferred simultaneously and the precursor frequency of Tag pI-specific CD8$^+$ T cells of each mouse was increased considerably. 5 d after transfer, draining lymph nodes (dLN) were isolated and analyzed for Tag-specific T cell proliferation indicated by CFSE dilution. Expression of the congenic marker CD45.1 enabled precise tracking of the transferred T cells in the isolated lymph node cell suspension. Cells of non-draining lymph nodes (ndLNs) from the opposite site of the mouse body were isolated as controls. No dilution of CFSE in form of decreased fluorescence was detected within the T cell population isolated from dLNs. This demonstrated that TCR-I T cells did not proliferate and thus, did not recognize the inoculated cancer cells when TagLuc was switched off. Confirming that transferred T cells in principle can be activated by TagLuc expressed on inoculated cancer cells, T cell proliferation in mice which had received TagLuc expressing cancer cells (clone 4 or TTC #3055 'on dox') was analyzed. T cells isolated from dLNs showed a distinct proliferation with up to 7 cell divisions being visible in the CFSE histogram as number of peaks (Fig. 3.13A. upper row, plot 2 and 4 from left side).

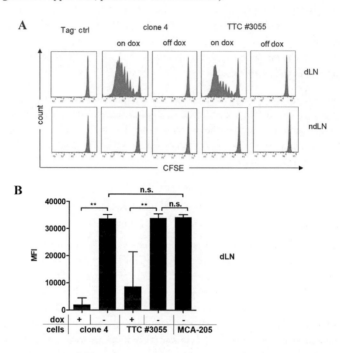

Figure 3.13 Cancer cells 'off dox' were not recognized by Tag pI-specific CD8+ T cells *in vivo*
(A) T cell proliferation in response to inoculated cancer cells was tested *in vivo*. CM2 mice were inoculated s.c. with 1×10^5 cancer cells (+ 10 mg/ml BD matrigel™) and co-injected i.v. with 1.9×10^6 CFSE-labelled CD8+Vβ7+ SV40-TCR-I transgenic splenocytes (CD45.1+). After 5 d draining lymph nodes (dLN) were analyzed for specific T cell proliferation by flow cytometry. As controls, non-draining lymph nodes (ndLN) of individual mice were analyzed as well. Shown is CFSE dilution as parameter for T cell proliferation (gate: CD8+CD45.1+ lymphocytes) for one representative mouse inoculated with clone 4 cancer cells per group (n=5). Tag⁻ cell line: MCA-205. **(B)** Mean flourescence intensity (MFI) of isolated CFSE labelled CD8+ lymphocytes did not decrease in dLNs of CM2 mice inoculated with clone 4 or TTC #3055 cancer cells 'off dox'. Results shown as MFI of CFSE ± SEM for 5 mice per group. Statistical analysis: two-tailed Mann-Whitney test with ** $p < 0.01$, not significant (n.s.) $p > 0.05$.

In order to quantify T cell proliferation in dLNs, the mean fluorescence intensity (MFI) of CFSE detected by flow cytometry was determined for each sample. MFI of T cells isolated from dLNs of mice inoculated with cancer cells 'off dox' was as high as MFI of T cells isolated from control mice that received Tag^- MCA-205 cells (Fig. 3.13B). Only T cells isolated from dLNs, but not from ndLNs of mice that were inoculated with cancer cells 'on dox' (Tag^+), showed a strong decrease in MFI.

Next, the kinetic of tumor cell rejection in CM2 mice that had or had not already developed Tag-specific T cell immunity was investigated to confirm the finding from the previous experiment. A slow rejection of TagLuc expressing cancer cells upon challenge would indicate a primary immune response whereas a fast rejection would indicate a secondary, so-called memory immune response. Therefore, CM2 mice were inoculated with clone 4 cancer cells that cultured 14 d without dox to switch off TagLuc expression. In one group ('immune'), TagLuc was directly induced by dox administration and all mice consequently rejected the inoculated clone 4 cancer cells. Furthermore, these mice developed Tag-specific $CD8^+$ T cells (data not shown) and later may more rapidly reject TagLuc-expressing cancer cells upon challenge. In the other group of mice ('naïve'), TagLuc was never induced in inoculated clone 4 cancer cells. Thus, no Tag-specific T cells were induced and T cells in these mice should have remained naïve. 56 d after TagLuc induction within the 'immune' group, mice of both groups were challenged s.c. with $3x10^6$ Tag-expressing Tet-TagLuc cancer cells and kinetic of their rejection was monitored by BL imaging. Mice of the 'immune' group rejected cancer cells completely until 6 d post challenge (d 4 and d 5 were not analyzed), whereas rejection by mice of the 'naïve' group was completed not before 9 d (Fig. 3.14). That significant difference in rejection kinetic strongly indicates that the Tag-specific immune response observed in the 'naive' group was a primary response upon first antigen recognition rather than a secondary immune response. Further, these results corroborate the assumption that, in general, T cell responses observed in the presented model were generated *de novo* after induction of TagLuc in resting cancer cells.

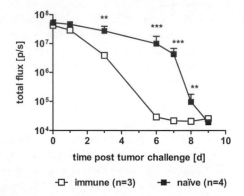

Figure 3.14 Slower rejection of TagLuc⁺ cancer cells upon challenge when TagLuc was never induced in resting clone 4 cancer cells

BL signal of CM2 mice inoculated with 3×10^6 Tet-TagLuc cancer cells s.c. is displayed. Previously, 'immune' and 'naïve' CM2 mice were inoculated with 1×10^5 clone 4 cancer cells 'off dox' at the contralateral site. CM2 mice from the 'immune' group (n=3) received dox to induce TagLuc expression, CM2 mice from the 'naïve' group (n=4) were left untreated. Tumor challenge with Tet-TagLuc cancer cells was performed 56 d after cancer cell inoculation and TagLuc induction. Shown are means ± SEM. Statistical analysis: unpaired, two-tailed t-test with *** $p < 0.005$, ** $p < 0.01$.

In summary, potential minimal TagLuc expression on cancer cells 'off dox' did not induce a specific T cell response upon inoculation in the described transplantation model. This finding was strengthened by the results from the *in vitro* T cell antigen recognition assay in which direct co-culture of Tag-specific TCR-I T cells with cancer cells 'off dox' likewise did not induce T cell activation (Fig. 3.6A, B).

3.2.7 Old mice still rejected TagLuc⁺ clone 4 cancer cells and developed a Tag-specific CD8⁺ T cell response

The data shown in Fig. 3.8 and Fig. 3.9 suggest that expression of TagLuc under non-inflammatory, resting conditions leads to a spontaneous CD8⁺ T cell response in immunocompetent CM2 mice. Mice used in the experiments described in the sections before were 10 and 20 weeks of age. During that age effective immune responses towards antigens e.g. expressed on cancer cells, can be mounted. In contrast, old mice lose the capability to reject transplanted tumor cells and have decreased T cell effector functions (Flood et al., 1981; Lustgarten et al., 2004). Schreiber et al. published in 2012 that only spleen cells from young, immunized mice rejected large, established tumors expressing a mutant peptide. Even though frequency of mutant peptide-specific T cells were equal compared to young mice, spleen cells from old, immunized mice, but also young, naïve mice, failed to reject tumors (Schreiber et al., 2012). It has been demonstrated in humans that incidence of cancer increases with age (Armitage and Doll, 1954) and it has been argued that this is a contribution of comprised immunity (reviewed in Derhovanessian et al., 2008). Therefore, it was asked next whether old CM2 mice can still reject clone 4 cancer cells when TagLuc is induced under resting conditions. Clone 4 cancer cells 'off dox' were inoculated into CM2 mice aged between 18 to 22 months to explore the impact of immunosenescence on $CD8^+$ T cell responses observed in this model. When TagLuc was induced by dox administration, a BL signal was detected in all young CM2 mice but only 75 % old mice. The reduced survival of inoculated cancer cells in old mice was most likely related to the age (Beheshti et al., 2015). In consequence, old CM2 mice in which TagLuc was not inducible after 4 weeks, were excluded from the experiment. Furthermore, it must be noted that 3 out of 9 mice from the group of old CM2 mice and 3 out of 4 mice from the group of young CM2 mice were albino and had a white fur. The different colored fur had influence on the sensitivity of minimal BL signal detection, which is generally lower in black furred mice compared to white-furred mice (Buschow et al., 2010). However, 4 d post TagLuc induction, a BL signal at the inoculation site was detected in all mice independent of fur color (Fig. 3.15A, B). A complete BL signal loss until 2 weeks post oncogene induction was observed in all young CM2 mice, whereas complete BL signal loss in old CM2 mice was detected 2 to 7 weeks post TagLuc induction (Fig. 3.15A, B).

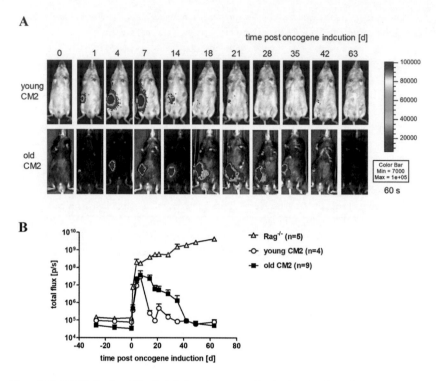

Figure 3.15 Old CM2 mice still rejected clone 4 cancer cells after TagLuc induction under resting conditions

(A) Kinetic of BL signal in old and young CM2 mice. $1x10^4$ clone 4 cancer cells in 10 mg/ml BD Matrigel™ were inoculated s.c. into mice. TagLuc was induced 27 d later by dox administration. One representative mouse is shown for each group. Young CM2: n=4, old CM2 n=9. (B) BL signal over time is displayed for each group inoculated with $1x10^4$ clone 4 cells. Results from one experiment are shown (± SEM).

Analysis of peripheral blood revealed an induction of Tag pI- and Tag pIV-specific $CD8^+$ T cells in young mice as well as in old mice. The time point of T cell appearance correlated with the observed decrease in BL signal (Fig. 3.15). In general, frequencies of both Tag-specific T cell populations were lower in old than in young CM2 mice (Fig. 3.16).

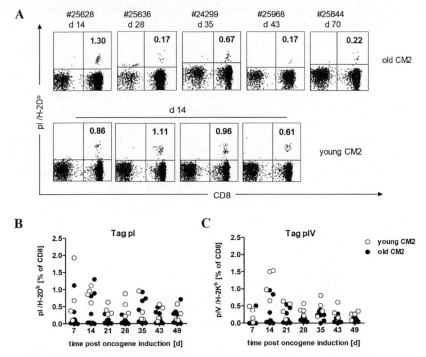

Figure 3.16 TagLuc expression in resting clone 4 cancer cells induced a Tag-specific CD8[+] T cell response in old CM2 mice

(A) Detection of Tag pI-specific T cells in peripheral blood of young (lower row) and old (upper row) CM2 mice by flow cytometry is displayed. Dot plots show the maximum frequency of Tag pI-specific CD8[+] T cells detected in individual mice at the indicated time point post TagLuc induction. Blood samples were stained with anti-CD3 and anti-CD8 antibody, and specific tetramer (Tag pI/H-2D[b]). Dot plots are shown for each young CM2 mouse and for 5 out of 9 old CM2 mice. Frequency of Tag pI/H-2D[b] tetramer[+] CD8[+] T cells is depicted. Gate: CD3[+] lymphocytes. **(B, C)** Kinetic of Tag pI-specific (B) and Tag pIV-specific (C) CD8[+] T cell populations is shown over time post TagLuc induction. Percentage of p/MHC tetramer[+] cells out of CD8[+] lymphocytes is shown. Black, open circles: young CM2 (n=4); black, filled circles: old CM2 (n=9).

In summary, these results show that rejection of TagLuc expressing cancer cells by newly induced Tag-specific CD8[+] T cells under resting conditions was independent of an aged immune system. However, kinetics of cancer cell rejection and T cell expansion were slower in old mice and might be potentially caused by the general immunosenescence in those mice.

3.2.8 Low TagLuc expression on clone 3D3 cancer cells induced Tag-specific CD8[+] T cells and resulted in regression of cancer cells

For elimination of cancer cells by T cells, a sufficient presentation of the tumor antigen through MHC molecules is necessary for initial T cell activation *in vivo*. Tumor antigens can be presented directly by cancer cells or indirectly by cross-presenting them on non-tumor cells (Bai et al., 2001). However, in both pathways the amount of presented antigen on the cell surface is critical for T cell activation (Morgan et al., 1999). The cancer cells used in the presented model express the tumor antigen (and oncogene) TagLuc, which is likely to be expressed at relatively high levels. Addressing the question whether lower TagLuc expression by cancer cells will also lead to CD8[+] T cell induction and cancer cell rejection in the proposed model, a single cell clone, named clone 3D3 (for further information see Appendix) was selected.

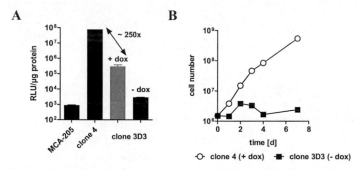

Figure 3.17 Clone 3D3 cancer cells expressed substantially less TagLuc protein and proliferated slowly upon dox deprivation

(A) Luciferase activity in clone 3D3 cancer cells 'on dox' and 'off dox' was compared to clone 4 cancer cells. After culture of the cancer cells in the presence or absence of dox, 1×10^6 cells (duplicates) were analyzed for luciferase activity. Cells were harvested, protein concentration was determined, and luciferase activity was measured as relative light units (RLU) in a luminometer (exposure time: 60 s). MCA-205: negative control. Results from 1 out of 2 experiments are shown as RLU ± SEM. (B) Doubling rate of clone 3D3 cancer cells cultured in the absence of dox compared to clone 4 cancer cells 'on dox'. 1.5×10^6 cells were seeded at d 0 and living cells were counted at the indicated time points.

Clone 3D3 cancer cells expressed ≈ 250 x less TagLuc than clone 4 cancer cells (Fig. 37A). Furthermore, clone 3D3 cancer cells grew independent of TagLuc expression, but TagLuc was still inducible via dox administration (Fig. 3.17A, B). The growth kinetic of clone 3D3 cancer cells 'off dox' was remarkably slower compared to clone 4 cancer cells 'on dox" (Fig. 3.17B). Considering the expected slow proliferation of clone 3D3 cancer cells *in vivo*, only 1×10^3 cells 'off dox' were inoculated into CM2 mice so that TagLuc will be induced in still a small number of cancer cells after a resting period of 4 weeks.

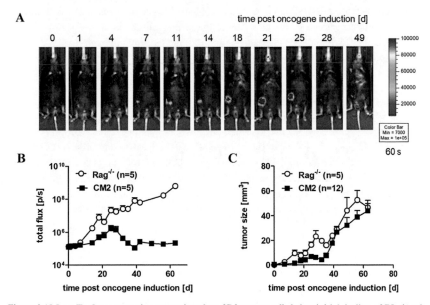

Figure 3.18 Low TagLuc expression on resting clone 3D3 cancer cells led to initial decline of BL signal but later outgrowth of tumors in CM2 mice
(A) BL signal kinetic of a CM2 mouse inoculated with 1×10^3 clone 3D3 cancer cells + 10 mg/ml BD Matrigel™ is shown. TagLuc was induced at 28 d post inoculation by dox administration and BL signals were detected by BL imaging. One representative mouse is shown from a two experiments (n=14). (B) BL signal over time is displayed for each albino Rag$^{-/-}$ (open circels) or albino CM2 mouse (black sqares) inoculated with 1×10^3 clone 3D3 cancer cells. BL signals of black CM2 mice are not displayed by the diagram. Results shown are representative for 1 out of 2 experiments with a total of n=10 Rag$^{-/-}$ and n=14 CM2 mice. Error bars correspond to SEM. (C) Tumor growth of clone 3D3 cells in Rag$^{-/-}$ and CM2 mice is shown for indicated number of mice. Results frome 1 out of 2 experiments are shown (± SEM).

Because clone 3D3 cancer cells slowly proliferated independent of TagLuc expression, a small tumor was palpable in 2 out of 5 Rag−/− mice and in 5 out of 12 CM2 mice 4 weeks post inoculation. Those tumors had volumes between 0,5 mm3 and 4 mm3, but no BL signal was detected at this site indicating no unintended TagLuc expression (Fig. 3.18A). TagLuc was induced by dox administration and a BL signal was subsequently detected in all mice. However, the time point of first BL signal detection varied between 1 and 25 d post TagLuc induction. On the one hand, these differences might be caused by different colored fur of the mice, that delayed detection of low BL signals in black mice. On the other hand, these differences might be caused by individual differences of each mouse in terms of cell survival and proliferation. BL signals detected in Rag−/− mice were slightly higher than those in CM2 mice but increased slowly over time in both groups (Fig. 3.18B)., BL signals in CM2 mice declined between 4 and 7 weeks post TagLuc induction, whereas they continued to increase over time in Rag$^{-/-}$ mice. Despite the obvious elimination of TagLuc expressing cancer cells, a low BL signal was still detected in few CM2 mice (Fig. 3.18B). However, during the decrease of BL signal in CM2 mice, tumor volumes decreased as well implying a Tag-specific cancer cell elimination. It must be noted that tumors grew out slowly in all CM2 mice at later time points, thereby exhibiting a similar growth kinetic found in $Rag^{-/-}$ mice (Fig. 3.18C). The tumor growth illustrated in Fig. 3.17B clearly demonstrate that clone 3D3 cancer cells were not addicted to TagLuc expression so that pre-existing antigen-negative variants might have been selected and grew out as tumors later.

During time of BL signal decline, Tag-specific $CD8^+$ T cells were detected in peripheral blood of CM2 mice. Tag pI- and Tag pIV-specific $CD8^+$ T cells were observed first 21 d post TagLuc induction in one CM2 mouse (Fig. 3.19A), which had a distinct BL signal at the inoculation site. Complete rejection of TagLuc expressing cancer cells in this mouse occurred until 35 d post TagLuc induction. 28 d post TagLuc induction, 8 out of 11 CM2 mice had developed a Tag pI-specific $CD8^+$ T cell population (Fig. 3.19B); and at 35 d post TagLuc induction, 9 out of 11 CM2 had developed a Tag pIV-specific T cell population (Fig. 3.19C), respectively. Appearance of Tag-specific $CD8^+$ T cells in blood was a consequence of distinct TagLuc expression in all mice and was always followed by a BL signal decrease. Similar to experiments with clone 4 cancer cells, Tag pI-specific $CD8^+$ T cells were detected earlier than Tag pIV-specific $CD8^+$ T cells. However, frequencies of both T cells populations were equal and varied between 0,28 % and 1,1 % out of $CD8^+$ T cells (Fig. 3.19).

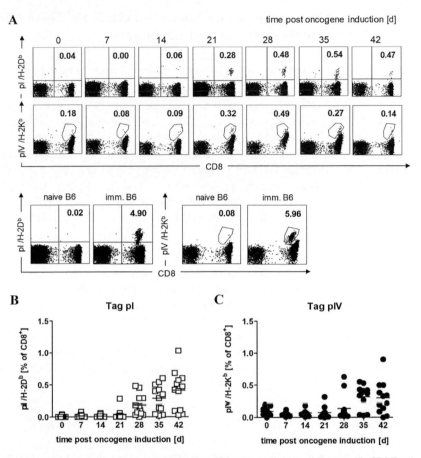

Figure 3.19 TagLuc expressed at low levels by clone 3D3 cancer cells induced Tag-specific CD8 T cells in CM2 mice

(A) Tag pI- and Tag pIV-specific CD8[+] T cells were stained in peripheral blood with corresponding specific p/MHC tetramer, monoclonal anti-CD3 and anti-CD8 antibodies before analysis by flow cytometry. Results of staining at indicated time points post TagLuc induction is shown for one representative CM2 mouse. The frequency of p/MHC tetramer[+] CD8[+] T cells is depicted in the plots. Gate: CD3[+] lymphocytes. Controls (lower panel): naïve B6 mouse (negative control) and B6 mouse immunized with Tet-TagLuc cancer cells ('imm. B6, positive control). **(B, C)** Frequencies of Tag pI- (B) and Tag pIV- (C) specific CD8[+] T cells in peripheral blood of CM2 mice is displayed over time. Vertical line shows mean of frequency of p/MHC tetramer[+] population (out of CD8[+] T cell population) detected at indicated time point post oncogene induction. Resuslts from 1 out of 2 independent experiments are shown (n=12).

3.3 Direct priming as a potential mechanism for induction of Tag-specific CD8[+] T cells in the absence of acute inflammation

3.3.1 Naïve TCR-I T cells were primed directly *in vitro* by TagLuc[+] cancer cells

There are two pathways how tumor antigens can induce activation and proliferation of naïve T cells: direct presentation by cancer cells or indirect presentation by antigen cross-presenting host cells. If T cells are primed by cancer cells directly, they need a so-called second signal which is usually provided by co-stimulatory molecules, such as B7.1 (CD80) and B7.2 (CD86), expressed predominantly on professional antigen presenting cells (APCs) (Freedman et al., 1991). Several groups published that only sufficient cross-presentation of tumor antigen results in an effective immune response (Otahal et al., 2005). In contrast, Ochsenbein et al. stated that CD8[+] T cells can be also primed in the absence of co-stimulatory signals, but co-stimulatory molecules enhance primed cytotoxic T cell responses in solid tumors (Ochsenbein et al., 2001).

It was asked whether T cells were primed directly by the cancer cells when TagLuc was induced. Therefore, clone 4 and TTC #3055 cancer cells were tested for expression of co-stimulatory molecules and their ability to stimulate naïve Tag-specific CD8[+] T cells *in vitro*. Both, clone 4 and TTC #3055 cancer cells showed no expression of the classical co-stimulatory molecules B7.1 or B7.2, whereas CY15 cancer cells (Kammertoens et al., 2005), which were used as a positive control, expressed both co-stimulatory molecules (Fig. 3.20A). However, staining of ICAM-1 (CD54) revealed a distinct expression of it on both cancer cell lines that was upregulated in the presence of IFN-γ (Fig. 3.20B) whereas B16F10 cells, which were used as a negative control, did not express ICAM-1.

Jenkinson et al. demonstrated that CD8[+] T cells can be directly activated by tumor cells independent of B7.1/B7.2 - CD28 binding but through ICAM-1/LFA-1 (lymphocyte function-associated antigen 1) interaction (Jenkinson et al., 2005). Since clone 4 and TTC #3055 cancer cells expressed ICAM-1, their ability to prime naïve TCR-I T cells was tested *in vitro*. TCR-I T cells were isolated from spleen of TCR-I transgenic mice and negatively sorted for CD44[−] (naïve) T cells. Co-culture of cancer cells with naïve TCR-I T cells resulted in T cell activation. This activation was characterized by expression of the early T cell activation marker CD69 and an increase in cell size, which led to a shift in the forward scatter (FSC) (Fig. 3.21B, C).

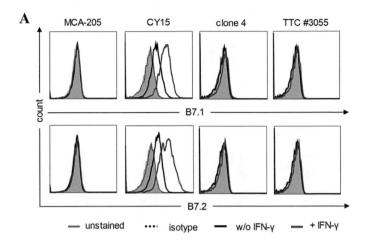

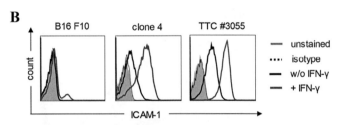

Figure 3.20 Expression of co-stimulatory molecule ICAM-1, but not B7.1 and B7.2 on clone 4 and TTC #3055 cancer cells

(A) Clone 4 and TTC #3055 cancer cells 'on dox' were cultured for 48 h in the presence or absence of IFN-γ (100 ng/ml) followed by staining with monoclonal anti-CD80 or anti-CD86 antibodies or isotype control antibodies. Expression of B7.1 and B7.2 was detected by flow cytometry. Negative control: MCA-205, positive control: CY15. Results shown are representative for 1 of 3 independent experiments. (B) Expression of ICAM-1 (CD54) on clone 4 and TTC #3055 cancer cells 'on dox'. After 48 h of culture, cells were stained with monoclonal anti-CD54 antibodies or isotype control antibodies. Negative control: B16 F10 melanoma cells. Results shown are representative for 1 of 2 independent experiments.

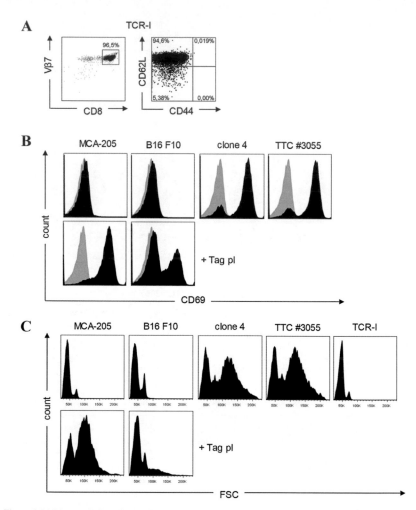

Figure 3.21 Direct priming of naïve TCR-I T cells *in vitro* by TagLuc⁺ cancer cells

(A) Spleen cells of a naïve TCR-I transgenic mouse were isolated and naïve CD8⁺ T cells were sorted with a purity of CD8⁺ Vβ7⁺ cells as indicated. Expression of CD62L and CD44 was detected by flow cytometry and is displayed for sorted CD8⁺ Vβ7⁺ population. Spleen cells were stained with monoclonal anti-CD8, anti Vβ7, anti-CD44 and anti-CD62L antibodies. **(B, C)** Clone 4 and TTC #3055 cancer cells were co-cultured with naïve TCR-I T cells for 3 d. Expression of activation marker CD69 on T cells (B) and change in T cell size (forward scatter, FSC) (C) were analyzed by flow cytometry (E:T ratio 10:1).T cells were stained with monoclonal anti-CD3, anti-CD8 and anti-CD69 antibodies. Gate: CD8⁺ Vβ7⁺ lymphocytes. Grey filled line: TCR-I T cells cultured without target cells. B16 F10 and MCA-205 cells were pulsed with 10^{-6} M Tag pI as positive control.

In addition, supernatants of the co-culture were analyzed in an IFN-γ ELISA. Only TCR-I T cells cultured with TagLuc⁺ cancer cells or TagLuc⁻ cancer cells that were exogenously loaded with Tag pI, produced substantial amounts of IFN-γ (Fig. 3.22). MCA-205 cells (no Tag expression) and B16F10 cells (no Tag and ICAM-1 expression) were used as negative controls and both only induced T cell activation and subsequent IFN-γ secretion when they were exogenously loaded with Tag pI (Fig. 3.21 and Fig. 3.22). It was an unexpected finding that B16F10 cells which do not express ICAM-1, also stimulated naïve TCR-I T cells when Tag pI was exogenously loaded onto the cells. However, compared to TagLuc-expressing clone 4 and TTC #3055 cancer cells, or MCA-205 cancer cells loaded with Tag pI, T cell activation caused by Tag pI-loaded B16F10 cells was less pronounced: up-regulation of CD69 and shift in FSC were lower.

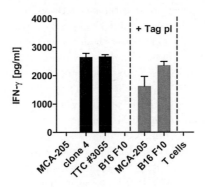

Figure 3.22 Directly primed TCR-I T cells produced IFN-γ in response to Tag pI expression by cancer cells

IFN-γ production of TCRI T cells after 3 d of co-culture was detected by ELISA (BD Biosciences). Results displayed are from a co-culture with an E/T ratio of 10:1. INF-γ concentration of undiluted supernatants is shown in [pg/ml] ± SEM. Results from one experiment.

These results suggest that direct priming of T cells through ICAM-1 expressed by cancer cells might play a role in the presented model. However, the frequency of TCR-I T cells in the *in vitro* assay was much higher than the frequency of Tag pI-specific T cells in naïve mice, and thus, the situation *in vivo* was not reflected accurately. Moreover, the results from B16F10 cancer cells which also induced T cell activation upon exogenous loading with peptide, implied that ICAM-1 was not solely responsible for priming of Tag-specific CD8⁺ T cells.

3.3.2 TCR-I T cells rejected TagLuc⁺ cancer cells in the absence of antigen cross-presentation by host cells

As already mentioned in the section before, cross-presentation plays an important role in initial activation of antigen-specific CD8⁺ T cells. It is described as an essential pathway leading to efficient priming of naïve CD8⁺ T cells *in vivo* (Huang et al., 1996). Cross-presentation can be found in the absence of secondary lymphoid tissues, but only if CD4⁺ T cell help is provided to the tumor antigen-specific T cells (Yu et al., 2003).

In order to investigate the role of cross-presentation and direct priming in activation of naïve CD8⁺ T cells, clone 4 cancer cells 'off dox' were inoculated into mice expressing mismatched MHC molecules. TCR-HAxRag$^{-/-}$/BALB/c mice are transgenic for a hemagglutinin-specific TCR restricted to MHC class I haplotype H-2^d (Morgan et al., 1996), and have no B cells. Those mice cannot cross-present the H-2D^b-restricted Tag epitope I and hence, were suitable to elucidate the role of direct T cell priming in this model. The use of T cell sufficient TCR-HAxRag$^{-/-}$/BALB/c mice as hosts was important to prevent antigen-unspecific, homeostatic expansion of transferred T cells and subsequent T cell activation, as it would occur in a T and B cell deficient host (Tanchot et al., 1997b). Rag$^{-/-}$ mice (MHC class I haplotype H-2^b, no B and T cells) and Rag$^{-/-}$/OT1 mice (MHC class I haplotype H-2^b, T cells express transgenic TCR specific for an epitope of ovalbumin) were used as controls. In both control mouse groups, Tag pI could be cross-presented to T cells by H-2D^b MHC class I molecules expressed on host cells, including APCs.

TagLuc expression was induced by dox administration 4 weeks after inoculation of 1x10⁴ clone 4 cancer cells 'off dox'. All mice showed a BL signal at the inoculation site 5 d post TagLuc induction and 1x10⁵ naïve TCR-I T cells were transferred at this time point. Before adoptive transfer, T cells were isolated from the spleen of naïve TCR-I transgenic mice and subsequently MACS-sorted for naïve CD44⁻ CD8⁺ T cells. BL signals post adoptive T cell transfer (ATT) were followed over time in each mouse and are shown in Fig. 21A for one representative mouse per group.

A BL signal loss at 7 d post ATT was observed in mice of both control groups, whereas in TCR-HAxRag$^{-/-}$/BALB/c mice a complete loss of BL signal was detected earliest 15 d post ATT (Fig. 3.23B, C). One mouse even rejected clone 4 cancer cells 50 d post ATT (Fig. 3.23C). Although rejection was remarkably later, adoptively transferred TCR-I T cells rejected TagLuc-expressing cancer cells independent of antigen cross-presentation by host cells (Fig. 3.23).

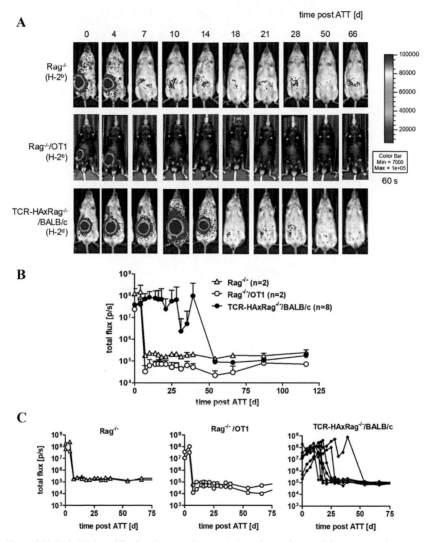

Figure 3.23 Re-induction of TagLuc in clone 4 cancer cells under resting conditions resulted in loss of BL signal in TCR-HAxRag$^{-/-}$/Balb/c mice

(A) BL signal kinetic of indicated mice is shown over time post ATT (d). Each mouse was inoculated with 1×10^4 clone 4 cancer cells (+ 10 mg/ml BD Matrigel^{TM}) that were oncogene deprived for 14 d *in vitro*. TagLuc was induced after 23 d by dox administration. 1×10^5 naïve (CD44$^-$) TCRI T cells were transferred 5 d post TagLuc induction. Mice shown are representative for each group (Rag$^{-/-}$, n=2, Rag$^{-/-}$/OT1, n=2, TCR-HAxRag$^{-/-}$/BALB/c, n=8). (B) BL signal kinetic over time (in d post ATT) is displayed for each group of mice. One Rag$^{-/-}$/OT1 mouse died before end of experiment (= 116 d post ATT). Displayed is total flux [p/s] ± SEM. (C) Individual BL signal kinetics of each mouse per group are shown at indicated time point post ATT (d).

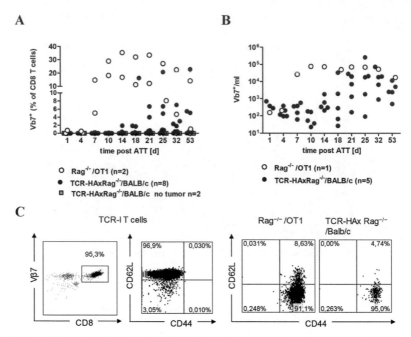

Figure 3.24 Expansion of transferred TCR-I T cells in the presence of TagLuc expressing cancer cells but absence of antigen cross-presentation
(A) Relative expansion of transferred T cells in peripheral blood is displayed over time (d post ATT). Cells were stained with anti-CD3, anti-CD8 and anti-Vβ7 antibodies and analyzed by flow cytometry. Gate: CD3⁺CD8⁺ lymphocytes. Open circles: Rag⁻/⁻/OT1 (n=2), black circles: TCR-HAxRag⁻/⁻/BALB/c (n=8). (B) Absolute numbers of transferred T cells were measured by use of Sphero™ AccuCount Particels (Spherotech). Peripheral blood was stained with monoclonal anti-CD3, anti-CD8 and anti-Vβ7 antibodies and counting beads were added directly before analysis in a flow cytometer. Gate: CD3⁺CD8⁺ lymphocytes. Open circles: Rag⁻/⁻/OT1 (n=1), black circles: TCR-HAxRag⁻/⁻/BALB/c (n=5). (C) Additional staining of peripheral blood cells shown in (A) with monoclonal anti-CD62L and anti-CD44 antibodies 14 d post ATT. Gate: CD8⁺ Vβ7⁺ lymphocytes. One representative plot from one mouse per group is displayed (Rag⁻/⁻/OT1: n=2, TCR-HAxRag⁻/⁻/BALB/c: n=5). First 2 plots show MACS-sorted TCR-I T cells before ATT. Second plot: peripheral blood cells gated on Vβ7⁺ CD8⁺ cells.

The transferred TCR-I T cells expanded simultaneously with the decreasing BL signals in TCR-HAxRag⁻/⁻/BALB/c mice. Analyzing peripheral blood revealed expansion of T cells earliest 18 d ATT in TCR-HAxRag⁻/⁻/BALB/c mice, whereas T cell expansion in Rag⁻/⁻ /OT1 mice was already detected 7 d post ATT (Fig. 3.24). Using special counting particles for flow cytometry absolute numbers of transferred T cells in peripheral blood were determined. TCR-I T cells in TCR-HAxRag⁻/⁻/BALB/c mice expanded up to 5x10⁶ cells per milliliter (ml) blood (25 d post ATT). Thus, absolute T cell expansion in these mice was similar to expansion observed in Rag⁻/⁻ /OT1 mice which also exhibited up to 5x10⁶ TCR-I T cells per ml blood (Fig. 3.24B). In addition, expanded T cells expressed CD44 indicating transition of the transferred T cells from a naïve into an effector memory phenotype (Fig. 3.24C).

Although T cell expansion was delayed in mice without the ability to cross-present antigens, the strength of T cell response was unaffected. Taken together, these data suggest that naïve TCRI T cells were directly primed by TagLuc-expresssing cancer cells in the absence of antigen cross-presentation on host cells and in a context without acute inflammation. Moreover, induced T cell response resulted in a long-term rejection of TagLuc-expressing cancer cells, which was comparable to mice in which cross-presentation of antigens was possible. Nevertheless, it cannot be excluded that unintended, nominal transfer of non-T cells, i.e. dendritic cells or monocytes, contributed to cancer cell rejection. However, there is little evidence, that these cells survive in such few numbers in a host with a mismatched MHC haplotype (Kirberg et al., 2001).

3.3.3 Naïve Tag-specific CD8$^+$ T cells expanded and rejected TagLuc$^+$ cancer cells in the absence of CD4$^+$ T cell help

CD8$^+$ T cells are central players of anti-tumor immunity and can eradicate tumor cells through their cytolytic activity (Martinez-Lostao et al., 2015). This is supported by the finding that most tumors express MHC class I molecules presenting tumor antigens to CD8$^+$ T cells (Wolfel et al., 1995; Boon and van der Bruggen, 1996), but no MHC class II molecules, and that CD8$^+$ T cells can be activated by direct recognition of peptide presented on MHC class I molecules (Ochsenbein et al., 2001; Wolkers et al., 2001). Further, adoptive transfer of CD8$^+$ T cell lines or clones have been shown to induce tumor regression in mouse models and human patients (Hanson et al., 2000; Ryan et al., 2001; Dudley et al., 2002; Anders et al., 2011; Robbins et al., 2013; Leisegang et al., 2016). However, there is evidence that tumor-reactive CD4$^+$ T cells can also contribute to anti-tumor immunity (Mumberg et al., 1999; Qin and Blankenstein, 2000; Corthay et al., 2005; Quezada et al., 2010; Tran et al., 2014). In addition, CD4$^+$ T cells are shown to be important for priming of cytotoxic CD8$^+$ T cells (Keene and Forman, 1982; Antony et al., 2005; Church et al., 2014).

In the following experiment, the role of CD4$^+$ T cells in developing a CD8$^+$ T cell response and subsequently rejecting TagLuc$^+$ clone 4 cancer cells was explored. Addressing this, splenocytes from naïve, transactivator-tolerant CM2 mice were isolated, subjected to MACS-depletion of CD4$^+$ T cells (Fig. 3.25) and 1x10^6 CD8$^+$ T cells were adoptively transferred into mice, which were inoculated with clone 4 cancer cells 'off dox' two weeks before. The use of P14xRag$^{-/-}$ as recipients, which also have endogenous CD8$^+$ T cells, was necessary to prevent antigen unspecific, homeostatic expansion and activation of transferred CD8$^+$ T cells (Tanchot et al., 1997b).

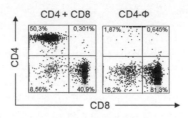

Figure 3.25 CD4⁺ T cell depletion of naïve CM2 splenocytes

Splenocytes from naïve CM2 mice were isolated and either depleted of CD4⁺ T cells by MACS ('CD4-Φ') or left untreated ('CD4+CD8'). Frequency of CD4⁺ T cells in both splenocytes suspensions was quantified by flow cytometry using monoclonal anti-CD3, anti-CD4 and anti-CD8 antibodies and is displayed as dot plot (gated on CD3⁺ lymphocytes).

TagLuc was induced in resting clone 4 cancer cells by dox administration at the same time point when CD4⁺ T cell-depleted splenocytes or undepleted control splenocytes were adoptively transferred into P14xRag⁻/⁻ mice. Regardless of CD4⁺ T cell depletion, all P14xRag⁻/⁻ mice that underwent adoptive cell transfer (ACT), rejected TagLuc-expressing clone 4 cancer cells (Fig. 3.26). Only one mouse that received CD4-depleted splenocytes, did not reject the cancer cells suggesting that a Tag-specific precursor CD8⁺ T cell may not have been contained within the 1x10⁶ transferred CD8⁺ T cells.

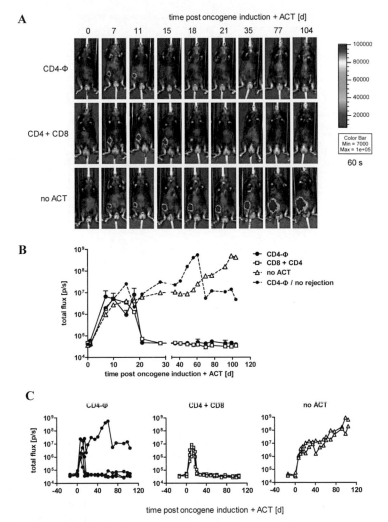

Figure 3.26 Rejection of TagLuc⁺ cancer cells in the absence of CD4⁺ T cells

(A) BL signal kinetic of indicated P14xRag$^{-/-}$ mice is shown over time post ACT (d). Each P14 xRag$^{-/-}$ mouse was inoculated with 1x10^4 clone 4 cancer cells (+ 10 mg/ml BD Matrigel^{TM}) that were oncogene deprived for 2 weeks before inoculation. TagLuc was induced after 14 d by dox administration and the indicated CM2-derived splenocyte suspension, each consisting of 1x10^6 CD8$^+$ T cells, was transferred i.v.. Mice shown are representative for each group (CD4-Φ, n=4, CD4+CD8, n=3, no ACT, n=2). Results from one out 2 experiments are shown. (B) BL signal kinetic over time (in d post ACT) is displayed for each group of mice. Displayed is total flux [p/s] ± SEM. One mouse of group 'CD4-Φ' did not reject clone 4 cancer cells and therefore, it is shown separately (black circle, dashed line). (C) Individual BL signal kinetics of each mouse per group are shown at indicated time point post ACT (d). Results from one out of 2 independent experiments are shown. Results of a second experiment are displayed in the 'Appendix' section.

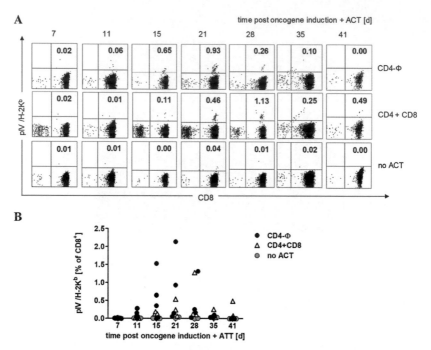

Figure 3.27 Expansion of transferred, naïve Tag pIV-specific CD8⁺ T cells upon TagLuc expression by cancer cells in the absence of CD4⁺ T cells

(A) Relative expansion of Tag pIV-specific CD8$^+$ T cells in peripheral blood of P14xRag$^{-/-}$ mice is displayed over time (in d post ACT, upper row). Cells were stained with monoclonal anti-CD3 and anti-CD8 antibodies, and p/MHC tetramer loaded with Tag pIV. Analysis was performed with a flow cytometer. Results of staining at indicated time point is shown for one representative P14xRag$^{-/-}$ mouse per group. (B) Frequency of Tag pIV-specific CD8$^+$ T cells is shown for each P14xRag$^{-/-}$ mouse at indicated time points (d post ACT). Gate: CD3$^+$ lymphocytes. Black, filled circles: CD4-Φ (n=4); black, open triangles: CD4+CD8 (n=3); grey, filled circles: no ACT (n=2). Results from one out of 2 independent experiments are shown.

During the time of rejection, an induction and expansion of Tag pIV-specific CD8$^+$ T cells was detected in peripheral blood of all mice (Fig. 3.27A, B). Despite the slightly earlier cancer cell rejection and induction of Tag-specific CD8$^+$ T cells in P14xRag$^{-/-}$ mice that received CD4$^+$ T cell-depleted splenocytes ('CD4-Φ'), also frequency of Tag pIV-specific CD8$^+$ T cells was overall higher in those mice compared to mice that received splenocytes comprising CD4$^+$ T cells ('CD4 + CD8'). The observed delay in induction of Tag-specific CD8$^+$ T cells might be explained by the concomitant transfer of regulatory CD4$^+$ CD25$^+$ T cells (T$_{reg}$). Those T$_{reg}$ cells are described to suppress anti-tumor responses (Shimizu et al., 1999).

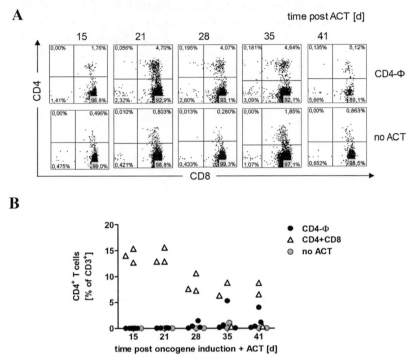

Figure 3.28 Rare, transferred CD4+ T cells did not expand during rejection of TagLuc+ cancer cells
(A) Frequency of CD4+ T cell in peripheral blood of P14xRag−/− mice was detected by flow cytometry and is displayed for each indicated time point and representative mouse (lower row, same mice also presented in Fig. 3.26A and Fig. 3.27A). Cells were stained with monoclonal anti-CD3, anti-CD4 and anti-CD8 antibodies. All depicted cells were detected within the CD3+ lymphocyte gate. **(B)** Frequency of CD4+ T cells is plottet for each individual mouse over time (d post ACT). Only one P14xRag−/− mouse of group 'CD4-Φ' showed a distinct expansion of rare, transferred CD4+ T cells. Gate: CD3+ lymphocytes. Black, filled circles: CD4-Φ (n=4); black, open triangles: CD4+CD8 (n=3); grey, filled circles: no ACT (n=2). Results from 1 out of 2 independent experiments are shown.

Since the transferred, CD4+ T cell-depleted splenocyte suspension still contained ~2 % CD4+ T cells (Fig. 3.25), unintended expansion of transferred CD4+ T cells was monitored over time post ACT. During the time of cancer cell rejection – between d 7 and d 18 post ACT – no expansion of CD4+ T cells was observed in peripheral blood of P14xRag−/− mice (Fig. 3.27A, B). Later, only one P14xRag−/− mouse had a substantial expansion of CD4+ T cells up to ~ 5 % (Fig. 3.27B). However, the P14xRag−/− mouse, which has not rejected the clone 4 cancer cells (Fig. 3.26C), had no expansion of CD4+ T cells. Therefore, one can argue that rare, transferred regulatory CD4+ T cells that may have suppressed potential anti-tumor responses, were unlikely to be the reason for continued progression of clone 4 cancer cells in this mouse.

In summary, these results demonstrate that Tag-specific CD8$^+$ T cells recognized TagLuc on clone 4 cancer cells and rejected them in the absence of CD4$^+$ T cell help. Presence or absence of CD4$^+$ T cells strikingly did not influence the rejection kinetic indicating that help provided by CD4$^+$ T cells did not play an indispensable role in priming and activation of Tag pIV-specific CD8$^+$ T cells in this model.

4 Discussion

In this study a novel transplantation model was established, and the interaction of cancer cells and T cells was studied to answer the century-old question whether immune surveillance against neoantigens expressed by transformed cells exists or not. The two cancer cell lines used herein conditionally expressed TagLuc as the cancer-driving oncogene and antigen. TagLuc expression required the presence of an active transactivator which was induced by dox administration in the described model. Further, Tag comprises MHC class I-restricted T cell epitopes that enabled the analysis of CD8[+] T cell responses in C57BL/6 mice. Although it originates from Simian virus 40, Tag was used as a model oncogene without viral or inflammatory context in this study. It mediates cellular transformation based on interaction with tumor suppressor proteins of which p53 and Rb are the most important.

4.1 A cancer transplantation model for studies of *de novo* T cell responses against neoantigens expressed in the absence of acute inflammation

4.1.1 Requirements of an appropriate cancer transplantation model

Whether the immune system can recognize and eliminate arising cancer cells is a subject of hot debates among scientists since more than 100 years. Different approaches and experimental systems have been utilized to answer this question. However, until now, not a single, adequate mouse model exists that simulates sporadic tumor formation accurately and thus, enables studying immune responses against newly expressed antigens as they might occur in humans. A suitable model to analyze cancer immune surveillance would have to comprise the following features: (1) expression of a tumor-specific antigen, (2) adjustable expression of the tumor-specific antigen in a spatio-temporal manner, (3) expression of the tumor-specific antigen in as few cells as feasible, (4) slow progression of transformed cells to tumors as it occurs in human sporadic cancer and (5) ability to precisely analyze tumor-specific immune responses, e.g. through cancer cell-specific expression of known MHC-restricted T cell epitopes.

Tumor transplantation is a widely applied experimental approach to follow the induction of immune responses and potential rejection of cancer cells. By using transplantation models, it is important to consider the findings by Schreiber et al. who clearly demonstrated by histological examination of cancer cell inoculums that an acute inflammation accompanied by immune cell infiltration is found within the first two weeks post subcutaneous inoculation (Schreiber et al., 2006; Schietinger et al., 2013). Together with the abundant cell death and subsequent antigen release, the inflammation-induced infiltration of immune cells can result in unintended recognition of the cancer cells.

4.1.2 Suitability of cancer cells expressing Tet system-regulated TagLuc

An initial objective of this study was to establish a cancer transplantation model that overcomes the limitations described beforehand thereby being suitable to study *de novo* immune responses in the absence of acute inflammation. Using TagLuc as the cancer-driving oncogene in our model, two important criteria were fulfilled: First, Tag is a true tumor-specific antigen with no homology in mice and thus, T cells were not tolerized against TagLuc. Second, Tag is demonstrated to elicit specific CD8$^+$ T cell responses against multiple epitopes in B6 mice with a H-2^b MHC haplotype (Mylin et al., 1995; Mylin et al., 2000) so that Tag-specific T cell responses can be studied. The fusion of Tag to Luc enabled visualization of tumor antigen expression *in vivo* but immune responses to Luc could have interfered with potential Tag-specific immune responses. Limberis et al. identified a H-2D^b-restricted CD8$^+$ T cell epitope of luciferase. However, T cell responses were rather weak and only observed after stimulation with high antigen amounts suggesting that luciferase is unlikely to elicit a CD8$^+$ T cell response in the presented model (Limberis et al., 2009). This is strengthened by the skin graft experiments published by Anders et al. in which Luc was not a rejection antigen in immunocompetent mice (Anders et al., 2011).

The applied cancer cell lines exhibited a tightly, Tet-regulated oncogene/antigen expression and allowed exclusion of unintended antigen recognition during the time of transplantation-induced inflammation. This feature was derived from an unexpected observation. As one would expect, the absence of dox led to inactivation of TagLuc expression. Since TagLuc is the cancer-driving antigen, its inactivation resulted in a strong decrease of proliferation. However, about one out of 4 cancer cells strikingly survived TagLuc deprivation and arrested in a status commonly found for senescent cells. A similar phenomenon is observed upon chemotherapy of human cancers or oncogene inactivation in experimental mouse cancer models (Bellovin et al., 2013), which induced therapy-induced senescence (TIS) in cancer cells (Ewald et al., 2010; Fan and Schmitt, 2017). In contrast to TIS, that is characterized by a terminal arrest of the senescent cells, cancer cells used in the presented study re-entered the cell cycle upon renewed TagLuc induction and started to proliferate again. These results suggest a special type of cellular arrest, comprising many features of senescent cells, e.g. H3K9 trimethylation and expression of SA-β-galactosidase (Bringold and Serrano, 2000), but exhibiting the unique ability to re-enter the cell cycle. According to this phenomenon, the observed senescent-like cellular arrest differed from the 'classical' senescence. Based on the finding that cancer cells survived temporary inactivation of the cancer-driving antigen TagLuc, the transplantation model presented in this work allowed induction of TagLuc expression and subsequent cell proliferation in resting cancer cells at any time *in vivo*.

4.1.3 Advantages of cancer cell visualization by BL imaging

In the work presented here, kinetics of cancer cell growth and rejection were monitored and visualized by BL imaging. The simultaneous expression of Luc and Tag enabled a sensitive, spatio-temporal measure of tumor antigen and oncogene expression *in vivo*. Since the presented model aimed to mimic an early phase of sporadic tumorigenesis, it was pivotal to inoculate as less cancer cells as feasible that still can be detected and monitored *in vivo* by BL imaging. While in other transplantation models usually approximately 1 million cancer cells are inoculated, a closer approximation to early malignant lesions was achieved by inoculating between 1×10^3 and 1×10^5 cancer cells. These low cell numbers were still visualizable by BL imaging. In an optimal model, only one transformed cell would be inoculated and thus, it would ideally reflect the initial phase of tumorigenesis. However, longitudinal tracking and monitoring of such few cancer cells by non-invasive imaging techniques is not applicable. It is to be noted that experiments conducted within this study would not have been possible without Luc as a highly sensitive measure of oncogene/antigen expression during a phase of cancer development when a tumor would not yet be palpable.

4.1.4 Lack of recognition of cancer cells 'off dox' by CD8⁺ T cells

A further important requirement of the proposed transplantation model was exclusion of unintended antigen expression in resting cancer cells – when no tumor-specific antigen should be expressed – by naïve Tag-specific CD8⁺ T cells. Although the advanced transactivator rtTA2^S-M2 with less basal activity in the absence of dox has been used (Urlinger et al., 2000), a very low, but detectable TagLuc expression was observed upon oncogene inactivation by dox deprivation. However, it was clearly demonstrated that this residual TagLuc expression did not induce activation of Tag-specific CD8⁺ T cells *in vitro* and *in vivo*. Moreover, even when the precursor frequency of Tag pI-specific CD8⁺ T cells was increased by transfer of TCR-I T cells into naïve, immunocompetent mice, residual TagLuc expression by inoculated, resting cancer cells was not recognized by the transferred CD8⁺ T cells. In a report by Kang et al. immune surveillance of senescent cells that express oncogenic *Nras* (Nras^{G12V}) was described to limit liver cancer development (Kang et al., 2011). In contrast, oncogene-deprived clone 4 and TTC #3055 cancer cells exhibited a senescent-like arrest but surveillance of those senescent-like cancer cells was not observed in the presented model. TagLuc could always be induced in resting cancer cells several weeks post inoculation. The immune surveillance demonstrated by Kang et al. was caused by a continuous CD4⁺ T cell-dependent clearance of premalignant, senescent cells. In addition, ras-specific Type I CD4⁺ helper cells were detected by IFN-γ ELISpot (enzyme linked immune spot) assay. Noteworthy, data in this study were obtained from a mouse model that based on hydrodynamic injection of vectors encoding for oncogenic *Nras*. Thus, the oncogene was likely to be homogeneously expressed in many hepatocytes across the entire liver. However, this is unlikely to happen during sporadic cancer development. Hence, immune responses observed in this model may not necessarily reflect immune responses against a premalignant lesion occurring during early tumorigenesis of human cancers. Different to the report of Kang et al., the role of CD4⁺ T cells was not directly addressed by the *in vivo* T cell proliferation experiment mentioned beforehand because monospecific TCR-I T cells were transferred. However, experiments, including the *in vivo* T cell proliferation assay, were conducted in immunocompetent mice having a complete CD4⁺ and CD8⁺ T cell compartment. In summary, neither residual, very low TagLuc expression nor the senescence-like phenotype of the cancer cells upon dox deprivation caused unwanted immune recognition and rejection of them in immunocompetent hosts. Hence, the presented model was suitable to study *de novo* CD8[+] T cell responses after TagLuc induction in resting cancer cells

4.1.5 Convergence of the model to human sporadic cancer

Most tumor transplantation models barely reflect sporadic cancer as it occurs in humans (Schreiber et al., 2006; Wen et al., 2012) and thereby hardly allow to transfer conclusions drawn from such models to human cancer patients. As mentioned beforehand, the tumor antigen used in a model plays an important role when cancer-specific immune responses are subjects of analysis. A tumor-specific antigen harboring at least one MHC-restricted T cell epitope is favored. Nevertheless, the number of mutations found in human cancer is rather low (Alexandrov et al., 2013) and thus, reduces the probability that unique, immunogenic neoantigens are expressed. The tumor-specific, cancer-driving antigen Tag, which is fused to Luc, represents a rare class of antigens. It contains multiple epitopes that can be recognized by T cells because it consists of > 700 amino acids without any homology in humans or mice. Corresponding human antigens like Tag can be found in cancers with a high degree of genetic instability. Microsatellite instability (MSI) that results from impaired DNA mismatch repair causes a predisposition to mutations that can lead to different types of cancer, e.g. colon, gastric, ovarian and skin cancer. For example, MSI is found in 15 % of all colorectal cancers and − besides hereditary forms, e.g. Lynch syndrome − includes sporadic colon cancer. Mutations in coding repeat sequences of microsatellites can lead to a shift in the open reading frame which results in the translation of new, so-called frameshift peptides and proteins consisting of a new amino acid sequence (Maby et al., 2016). Those frameshift peptides can be immunogenic in human cancer patients (Saeterdal et al., 2001; Ishikawa et al., 2003; Reuschenbach et al., 2010; Maletzki et al., 2013). Hence, Tag in the presented model, reflects a neoantigen as it can be expressed by sporadic cancers with MSI. Moreover, immune responses observed in this model may recapitulate initial interactions between new arising cancer cells and the adaptive immune system in human cancer patients.

4.1.6 Limitations and prospects of the model

Although the model closely reflects sporadic cancer at an early stage of tumorigenesis and enables studying *de novo* immune responses against a tumor-specific antigen, also some limitations have to be mentioned. It is important to consider that the small number of cancer cells in which TagLuc can be expressed, is still higher compared to the natural situation. Sporadic cancer is the result of mutational events occurring in one single cell rather than in a couple of thousands cells (Hahn and Weinberg, 2002). However, the inoculation of only 1×10^3 cancer cells 'off dox' into immunocompetent hosts (Fig. 3.12) approached a situation found in early human sporadic cancer development. Considering the experimentally determined average *in vivo* survival rate of 10 % for this cancer cell line, TagLuc was induced in only 100 cells in the mentioned experiment. Theoretically, the presented model would even allow inoculation of only one single cancer cell, but with respect to the inoculation-induced cell death (Schreiber et al., 2006), very large groups of mice would be required. Moreover, the advantages of cancer cell visualization by BL imaging would be negated by the detection limit of the cancer cells.

Using Matrigel to promote survival of inoculated cancer cells conceivably led to a microenvironment which may not reflect milieus in human sporadic cancer. Cancer cells of a sporadic tumor are also embedded in extracellular matrix (ECM) (Lu et al., 2012) but composition of the ECM may depend on the site of tumor development and differ among different cancers. On the contrary, composition of the Matrigel used in the presented study can be considered as always similar when used in experiment. The commercially available Matrigel is derived from the murine Engelbreth-Holm-Swarm tumor, a chondrosarcoma producing a matrix resembling basement membranes (Orkin et al., 1977; Kleinman and Martin, 2005). Besides structural proteins such as laminin, collagen and proteoglycans, Matrigel also contains growth factors like tumor growth factor β (TGF-β) and epidermal growth factor (EGF) (Vukicevic et al., 1992; Hughes et al., 2010). These growth factors can promote proliferation of cancer cells or infiltration of immune cells into the Matrigel plug and thus, could have favored cancer cell recognition by the immune system after antigen induction. However, in a study by Plattner et al., empty Matrigel plugs have been analyzed by histology and only few infiltrating leukocytes were detected within (Plattner et al., 2013). In a vaccine study by Zhou et al., also exceedingly low numbers of infiltrating immune cells were detected within empty Matrigel plugs (Zhou et al., 2007), suggesting that application of Matrigel does not alter the microenvironment crucially. Nevertheless, to avoid any influence of Matrigel on the outcome of possible tumor-specific immune responses in the presented model, artificial basement membrane matrices, e.g. PuraMatrix® (Kim et al., 2007) would be an alternative option. In addition, *ex vivo* analyses of Matrigel-cancer cell plugs by immunohistochemistry or flow cytometry should be done to quantify potential infiltrating cells before antigen induction and hence, provide better estimation about preferential immune responses that may not be found without usage of Matrigel.

As mentioned already beforehand, cancer cells used in this work arrested in a senescent-like status before induction of TagLuc led to renewed proliferation. It has been shown that senescent cells develop a secretory phenotype (SASP) including secretion of interleukin (IL)-1 and IL-6. These interleukins can alter the microenvironment and hence, affect neighboring cells (Coppe et al., 2008; Rodier and Campisi, 2011). Inoculation of senescent cancer cells in this study could have altered the microenvironment and promoted attraction of immune cells to the inoculum. In contrast, some of the factors secreted by senescent cells create an immunosuppressive environment (Hinds and Pietruska, 2017) hampering potential immune responses. However, detailed analysis of the senescent-like status of cancer cells was not subject of investigation in this study.

In this study, cancer cells were inoculated subcutaneously (s.c.) and destructive T cell responses against TagLuc – a neoantigen expressed by the cancer cells – were observed. However, the skin is not only a physical barrier to invading pathogens, but also an immune organ regulating local immunity. Hence, T cell immunity detected in the presented model could have been influenced by the special immunological microenvironment in the skin but may be different in other organs with a different microenvironment. Primarily, skin-resident immune cells, such as Langerhans cells which function as professional APCs (Bennett and Chakraverty, 2012), and resident T cells (Zaid et al., 2014) might have influenced immune responses to TagLuc in the presented model. However, the subcutaneous tissue mainly contains monocytes and macrophages whereas a variety of DCs can be found in the dermis (Tong et al., 2015). DCs are the main immune cell subset involved in T cell priming but not frequently represented in the subcutaneous tissue. Thus, a greater immunogenicity of s.c. inoculated cancer cells was not expectable in the model herein. This is supported by a study of Joncker et al. as intradermal but not s.c. transplantation of tumors augmented immunogenicity and induced T cell-mediated rejection caused by recruitment of dermal DCs (Joncker et al., 2016). Contrastingly, skin DCs and Langerhans cells presenting antigens under so-called steady state conditions in the absence of inflammation, were shown to rather induce T cell tolerance than T cell-mediated immunity (Ohl et al., 2004). For the presented transplantation model this would mean that presentation of TagLuc in the draining lymph nodes by skin-derived DC and Langerhans cells would also have induced T cell tolerance since TagLuc was always expressed under non-acute inflammatory conditions. Consequently, immunocompetent host would not have rejected the cancer cells due to induced peripheral tolerance. However, the results of this study clearly demonstrate an effective CD8$^+$ T cell response in immunocompetent mice although the antigen TagLuc was presented in the absence of acute inflammation.

It is beyond doubt that the microenvironment influences tumor-specific immunity (Bissell and Radisky, 2001; Fridman et al., 2012; Gajewski et al., 2013). Thus, application of the presented model to other organs, such as pancreas, kidney or mammary fat pad would provide further insights into organ-dependent cancer immune surveillance.

4.2 Immune response to newly expressed TagLuc on cancer cells in the absence of acute inflammation

4.2.1 Spontaneous CD8$^+$ T cell responses against TagLuc expressed on cancer cells under resting conditions

The central question of this study was to investigate existence of immune surveillance of sporadic cancer by tumor-specific, cytotoxic CD8$^+$ T cells. Many models have been employed in the past to obtain data about anti-tumor T cells responses. In most of them the host is exposed to an artificially high number of cancer cells at a single time point, e.g. through conventional transplantation experiments or transgenic mouse cancer models with a tissue-specific oncogene/antigen expression. In other models, e.g. using chemicals to induce carcinogenesis, specific T cell responses cannot be analyzed because tumor antigens are unknown. Moreover, chemical carcinogenesis is shown to be influenced by non-specific inflammatory responses which may be altered in immunodeficient mice (Blankenstein and Qin, 2003). In other sporadic cancer models, oncogene activation is induced through Cre-mediated stop cassette deletion (Meuwissen et al., 2001) or by spontaneous recombination (Johnson et al., 2001). But antitumor immune responses have not been analyzed in those models and yet, they do not provide clear evidence for immune surveillance. The sporadic cancer model established in this study combines beneficial properties of transplantation models – expression of a specific tumor antigen by a defined cell population at a single time point at one body site – with the advantages of transgenic models. The latter is marked by tumor antigen expression and sporadic cancer development that are mostly induced conditionally under resting conditions and in the absence of acute inflammation. Moreover, the transplantation model exhibits only minimal mouse-to-mouse variances compared to transgenic mouse models (Willimsky and Blankenstein, 2005) and thus, facilitates simple and simultaneous investigations of T cell responses in large groups of mice. Furthermore, analyzing neoantigen-specific T cells responses in the primary host essentially requires that the tumor antigen is not expressed priorly by non-cancer cells, which is known to induce central T cell tolerance (Schwartz, 2003). This is an inherent problem of transgenic cancer models in which former transgene expression cannot be utterly excluded and may lead to central or peripheral T cell tolerance. Since recipient mice used in this study were not transgenic for TagLuc, previous, unwanted antigen expression by thymic epithelial cells was decidedly excluded. In consequence, TagLuc was a truly tumor-specific antigen and $CD8^+$ T cells were not subjected to self-tolerance in this model. Thus, the presented transplantation model has a great advantage over other tumor models and allows studying *de novo* T cell responses.

The role of adaptive immunity in controlling tumor outgrowth was demonstrated indirectly by the first experiments performed in immunodeficient $Rag^{-/-}$ mice. When TagLuc was induced in resting cancer cells, BL signals increased continuously and subsequently, tumors grew out within 2 to 3 months. Since $Rag^{-/-}$ mice do not have mature B and T cells (Mombaerts et al., 1992), these experiments illustrated that innate immunity was unable to prevent or control tumor outgrowth. Although NK cells, which are lymphocytes of the innate immune system, are present in $Rag^{-/-}$ mice and can potentially eradicate cancer cells, they did not have a crucial impact on tumor progression. Hence, it can be concluded that any effects on cancer cell progression observed in immunocompetent mice were likely caused by cells of the adaptive immune system. Albeit, synergistic effects of innate and adaptive immune cells which can take place in immunocompetent hosts, cannot be excluded.

Next, $CD8^+$ T cell responses against newly expressed TagLuc was investigated in immunocompetent CM2 mice. It was of outmost importance to exclude any kind of cancer cell recognition by the immune system before the cancer-driving, tumor-specific antigen TagLuc is induced experimentally by dox administration. Supported by the findings of this study that cancer cells 'off dox' were neither recognized *in vitro* nor *in vivo* by Tag-specific $CD8^+$ T cells in proliferation assays, it was an expected outcome that TagLuc expression in resting cancer cells was inducible in all CM2 mice. The assumption that inoculation of cancer cells 'off dox' do not evoke an unintended immune response was confirmed by staining of peripheral blood for Tag-specific $CD8^+$ T cells. Such Tag-specific T cells were not detectable at time points before TagLuc induction. In addition, CM2 mice that were inoculated with cancer cells 'off dox' but never experienced dox-mediated TagLuc induction, rejected a challenge with Tag-expressing tumor cells remarkably later compared to CM2 mice in which TagLuc was induced directly post s.c. inoculation before tumor challenge. These results corroborate that each immune response observed in CM2 mice upon TagLuc induction was most likely induced *de novo* and a so-called primary immune response. When analyzing peripheral blood of CM2 mice, Tag-specific CD8$^+$ T cells emerged between 10 and 14 days after TagLuc induction in resting cancer cells. In association with the observed BL signal loss during that time, this strongly indicates that newly induced CD8$^+$ T cells caused rejection of Tag-expressing cancer cells. These results are strengthened by the finding that no Tag-specific CD8$^+$ T cells were found before TagLuc induction. Hence, immune surveillance of cancer cells by CD8$^+$ T cells was demonstrated in a transplantation model that closely reflects sporadic cancer development. This observation is in strong contrast to a study by Willimsky et al. in which spontaneous activation of the dormant oncogene Tag in single cells induced T cell tolerance and no protection from tumor growth (Willimsky and Blankenstein, 2005). Although tumors were immunogenic and initially induced Tag-specific CD8$^+$ T cells, mice developed a T cell tolerance and tumors progressed. The same group later found out that T cell tolerance in this model was induced by premalignant lesions and paradoxically, was observed at the same time when Tag-specific antibodies were detected (Willimsky et al., 2008). However, in this model of stochastic oncogene activation it is unclear how many cells expressed Tag at which level during the lifespan of the host. Hence, one can only speculate if a single premalignant lesion would have also induced T cell tolerance. On the contrary, CD8$^+$ T cell responses observed in the presented model, were induced by a single cancer cell population at a single body site.

In this study, Tag-specific CD8$^+$ T cell populations recognizing two different epitopes were detected by p/MHC tetramer staining. CM2 mice developed functional T cell responses against the two prominent Tag epitopes described to be immunogenic in mice (Mylin et al., 1995; Mylin et al., 2000). The hierarchy of Tag-specific CD8$^+$ T cells found in this study differed from that found by group of Mylin. CD8$^+$ T cells specific for epitope I were found with marginal higher frequency than CD8$^+$ T cells specific for epitope IV and thus, hierarchy was conversed. This might be explained by the different modes of 'immunization'. In the study by Mylin et al., Tag-specific CD8$^+$ T cell responses were generated by repeated intraperitoneal injection of high numbers of Tag-transformed cells or intravenous injection of a recombinant vaccinia virus encoding for Tag/Tag epitopes. This ensures rapid delivery of high antigen amounts and partially already preprocessed epitopes, which creates ideal conditions for cross-priming by APCs. In contrast, overall amount of Tag or Tag epitopes presented by cancer cells in the presented model can be considered lower compared to immunization studies. Further, the absence of acute inflammation that always accompanies needle injection, may also alter the immune response to Tag. Textor et al. showed that processing of Tag epitope IV by the immunoproteasome is dependent on IFN-γ whereas processing of Tag epitope I is independent of IFN-γ (Textor et al., 2016). Since IFN-γ is a major cytokine contributing to inflammation, it is not expected to be present at high concentration during the time of tumor antigen expression, because TagLuc was always induced after the inoculation-induced acute inflammation was vanished. Consequently, the IFN-γ-independent Tag epitope I might be more abundantly expressed on the cancer cell surface than IFN-γ-dependent Tag epitope IV and hence, might have led to an altered hierarchy of emerging CD8$^+$ T cells.

4.2.2 Immune response to TagLuc in old mice

This study demonstrates that old mice can also reject TagLuc-expressing cancer cells under resting conditions. Tag-specific CD8$^+$ T cells were detected by p/MHC tetramers indicating a T cell-mediated rejection of the cancer cells as it was observed in young CM2 mice. These findings are contradicting to studies published by others. Transplanting ultraviolet light (UV)-induced tumors, Spellman and Daynes demonstrated that incidence of tumor susceptibility increases in old mice (Spellman and Daynes, 1978). Moreover, Flood et al. showed that the capability of mice to reject transplanted immunogenic fibrosarcoma cells decreases with increasing age of the recipient host (Flood et al., 1981). The impaired tumor rejection was explained by quantitative and qualitative changes of the immune response observed in aged mice. In a study by Schreiber et al., spleen cells from young, immunized mice rejected large tumors expressing a mutant peptide whereas spleen cells from old, immunized or young, naïve mice failed to reject tumors (Schreiber et al., 2012). In contrast, although slower and more diverse rejection kinetics and higher variations in frequency of Tag-specific CD8$^+$ T cells were observed, all old mice ultimately rejected TagLuc-expressing cancer cells in the model herein. The variation in rejection kinetics and T cell frequencies may indicate quantitative changes in the immune response but a qualitative change of it in old mice compared to young mice was not found.

In another study, transplantation of an immunogenic B cell lymphoma resulted in tumor progression in old mice, but not in young mice. Only if the co-stimulatory molecule B7.1 was expressed by the implanted lymphoma cells, the unresponsiveness in old mice was reverted and a protective immune response was elicited (Lustgarten et al., 2004). In contrast, cancer cells used in the study herein were demonstrated to not express co-stimulatory molecules but were still rejected by old mice. This indicates that rejection, observed in old mice was independent of classical co-stimulation provided by cancer cells in the presented model.

4.2.3 Immune response to cancer cells expressing low levels of TagLuc

It is of general acceptance that so-called regressor tumors are rejected by immunocompetent hosts because they express rejection antigens that can be recognized by T cells (Kripke, 1974; Ward et al., 1989). For an effective immune response and tumor rejection, high expression levels of tumor antigen are an essential requirement. It is on debate whether high levels of antigen expression directly prime T cells (Ochsenbein et al., 2001) or lead to enhanced cross-presentation by non-tumor cells and indirect priming of T cells (Ochsenbein et al., 2001; Spiotto et al., 2002). Independent of the potential mode of T cell activation, both cancer cell lines used in this study are regressor cell lines and were shown to be rejected by immunocompetent mice, even in the absence of acute inflammation. The rejection was accompanied by induction of Tag-specific CD8[+] T cells indicating sufficient expression of tumor antigen on the cancer cells. Both cancer cell lines expressed TagLuc at relatively high levels. Contrary to expectations, the cancer cell line clone 3D3, which expressed ~ 250-fold less TagLuc compared to clone 4 cancer cells, also induced Tag-specific CD8[+] T cells and subsequent cancer cell regression in immunocompetent mice. This result demonstrates that − even expressed at low levels − TagLuc levels were sufficiently high for priming of naïve CD8[+] T cells under resting conditions. Induction of Tag-specific CD8[+] T cells and cancer cell regression occurred notably later compared to clone 4 cancer cells. Contradicting to existing literature (Morgan et al., 1999; Spiotto et al., 2002), low levels of tumor antigen seemed to delay but not prevent priming of CD8[+] T cells in the presented model. In human tumors, antigen presentation is often decreased, e.g. through down-regulation of MHC molecules or proteins associated with antigen presentation. This may lead to reduced recognition of cancer cells by T cells (Vitale et al., 1998; van Houdt et al., 2008). In contrast, a decreased TagLuc expression by cancer cells used in this study did not alter immunogenicity. Moreover, frequencies of Tag-specific CD8[+] T cells detected in peripheral blood were comparable to frequencies detected when TagLuc was expressed at high levels on cancer cells. An explanation may be that different to most tumor antigens found in human patients, Tag comprises several MHC class I-restricted T cell epitopes which increases probability of T cell recognition even if presented at low levels. Once Tag-specific CD8[+] T cells were primed, they seemed to exhibit similar expansion and cytotoxic effector functions as CD8[+] T cells induced by cancer cells with high TagLuc expression. Because CD8[+] T cell-mediated rejection of clone 3D3 cancer cells was remarkably delayed compared to rejection of clone 4 cancer cells, another explanation might be reasonable. Dox-mediated TagLuc induction increased clone 3D3 cancer cell proliferation, which in turn resulted in more cancer cells that expressed TagLuc. As a consequence, the total amount of expressed TagLuc was sufficient to activate Tag-specific CD8[+] T cells. In conclusion, immune surveillance of TagLuc-expressing cancer cells was also found in cancerous lesions expressing low antigen amounts.

4.3 Direct priming of Tag-specific CD8[+] T cells

In the third part of this work, the potential mode of T cell activation was elucidated. It was questioned whether Tag-specific CD8[+] T cells are primed directly by cancer cells and whether CD4[+] T cells play a role in generating a cytotoxic T cell response.

4.3.1 Co-stimulatory molecules

Co-stimulation is believed to be inevitable for direct priming of CD8[+] T cells and their differentiation into cytotoxic effector cells (Linsley et al., 1991; Chen et al., 1993). Surface staining for expression of the classical co-stimulatory molecules B7.1 and B7.2 was negative for both cancer cell lines suggesting that direct priming of CD8[+] T cells is unlikely to happen. However, both cancer cell lines expressed ICAM-1, a surface glycoprotein with high affinity to LFA-1 expressed on leukocytes, e.g. CD8[+] T cells. In a study by Jenkins et al. it was reported that CD8$^+$ T cells were directly activated by tumor cells through ICAM-1/LFA-1 interaction (Jenkinson et al., 2005). Another study published by the same group also demonstrated the potential of ICAM-1 expressed by cancer cells as an alternative co-stimulatory molecule for priming of naïve CD8$^+$ T cells (Basingab et al., 2016). Results from the *in vitro* priming assay with naïve TCR-I T cells supports this hypothesis since TCR-I T cells were activated and secreted IFN-γ when they were cultured with ICAM-1-expressing cancer cell lines clone 4 or TTC #3055. In contrast, TCR-I T cells co-cultured with ICAM-1 negative cell lines that were exogenously loaded with Tag pI, exhibited a diminished activation profile. Nevertheless, the few studies reporting priming of naïve CD8$^+$ T cells via ICAM-1 expressed by cancer cells mainly investigated interactions *in vitro* and thus, relevance *in vivo* remains ambiguous.

4.3.2 Direct priming in tumor-draining lymph nodes

According to the data published by the group of Zinkernagel, direct priming of CD8$^+$ T cells is possible if tumor cells migrate to draining lymph nodes (LNs) at early time points and for sufficient duration (Ochsenbein et al., 2001). To test this hypothesis in the model herein, draining LNs from immunocompetent mice that have been inoculated with clone 4 cancer cells, were isolated 5 d post TagLuc induction for *ex vivo* culture. However, no clone 4 cancer cells that potentially have migrated to the draining LN, grew out (n=5, data not shown). Nevertheless, even if there is any migration of cancer cells, the expected number in draining LNs is supposed to be rather low. In consequence, it cannot be excluded that culture conditions were not optimal for survival of such few cells. Further efforts are required to prove whether cancer cells migrate to lymph nodes in this model thereby supporting the direct priming hypothesis.

4.3.3 Role of CD4$^+$ T cells in priming of Tag-specific CD8$^+$ T cells

In this study, a destructive Tag-specific CD8$^+$ T cell response was developed in the absence of CD4$^+$ T cells. When TagLuc expression was induced in clone 4 cancer cells under resting conditions, adoptively transferred, naïve CD8$^+$ T cells recognized TagLuc expressing cancer cells and expanded in P14xRag$^{-/-}$ mice. Moreover, absence of CD4$^+$ T cells did not alter rejection kinetics or development of Tag-specific CD8$^+$ T cells compared to mice that received CD8$^+$ T cells together with CD4$^+$ T cells. These results are in strong contrast to the findings of other research groups that reported an essential role of CD4$^+$ T cells in tumor rejection. For example, several studies imply the importance of CD4$^+$ T cell help for priming of cytotoxic CD8$^+$ T cells (Keene and Forman, 1982; Gao et al., 2002; Bos and Sherman, 2010). According to this, absence of CD4$^+$ T cells has been shown to diminish cytotoxic T cell responses (Antony et al., 2005) or to abolish tumor recognition and rejection (Greenberg et al., 1981; Tempero et al., 1998). However, mostly immune responses against self/tumor-associated antigens have been investigated in these studies. Thus, the found importance of CD4$^+$ T cells for induction of functional CD8$^+$ T cell responses may not apply to the presented model in which a tumor-specific antigen was expressed. In contrast to T cells recognizing tumor specific antigens, the precursor frequency of CD8$^+$ T cells recognizing tumor-associated antigens is expected to be low due to central tolerance mechanisms (Rizzuto et al., 2009). Therefore, CD4[+] T cell help may play an important role in induction of tumor-reactive T cell responses when tumor-associated antigens are expressed. CD8[+] T cells used in the corresponding experiment were derived from non-tolerant, naïve mice. Thus, the independency of tumor rejection from the presence of CD4[+] T cells can be explained by the fact, that the number and avidity of Tag-specific CD8[+] T cells was not reduced due to negative selection in the thymus. Consequently, T cell numbers were sufficient to be primed by TagLuc expressed on cancer cells *in vivo* and elicit a cytotoxic response.

Contrary to expectations, rejection kinetics did not differ considerably among mice that received CD4[+] T cell-depleted splenocytes and mice that received both, CD4[+] and CD8[+] T cells. One reason might be, that the depletion of CD4[+] T cells also included a removal of regulatory T cells (T_{regs}). Since T_{regs} are well described as an immunosuppressive cell population (Sakaguchi et al., 2010), they are also capable to suppress anti-tumor immune responses. In accordance with this, removal of T_{regs} has been demonstrated to induce tumor immunity (Onizuka et al., 1999; Shimizu et al., 1999). Therefore, absence of immunosuppressive T_{regs} may have compensated for the absence of CD4[+] T cell help in the described adoptive transfer experiment of this study. Consequently, kinetics of cancer cell rejection were comparable in the presence and the absence of CD4[+] T cells.

4.3.4 Role of cross-presentation in priming of Tag-specific CD8[+] T cells

Adoptive transfer of naïve TCR-I T cells into MHC-mismatched TCR-HAxRag$^{-/-}$/BALB/c mice resulted in rejection of TagLuc-expressing clone 4 cancer cells. This finding suggests direct priming of Tag-specific CD8[+] T cells by clone 4 cancer cells independently from antigen cross-presentation by professional APCs. Studies addressing antigen cross-presentation are controversially discussed among the scientific community. Results of those studies whether argue for or against the relevance of T cell cross-priming. The importance of cross-presentation for induction of antigen-specific T cell responses has been demonstrated by several research groups (Huang et al., 1994; Speiser et al., 1997; Nguyen et al., 2002; Chen et al., 2004). In contrast, the results from the adoptive transfer experiment in TCR-HAxRag$^{-/-}$/BALB/c mice illustrate that cross-presentation of Tag epitope I was not necessary for priming of naïve TCR-I T cells. Contrarily, TCR-I T cells could have been only primed directly in that experiment. Evidence for direct priming of tumor antigen-specific T cells was also found by other research groups (Kündig et al., 1995; Ochsenbein et al., 2001; Wolkers et al., 2001). As mentioned already before, direct priming of T cells is dependent on the migration of cancer cells to draining lymph nodes. A study by Pavelic et al. demonstrated that only direct priming of T cells induced an immune response against a subdominant epitope (Pavelic et al., 2009) implying the importance of direct antigen presentation for generating a polyspecific immune response. In contrast, Otahal et al. found that inefficient cross-presentation limits the immune response to a subdominant epitope of Tag (Otahal et al., 2005). Interestingly, it has been reported that different antigens are recognized through direct and cross-priming. For direct priming, ongoing antigen processing by cancer cells was required whereas cross-priming was independent from new processing of antigen

(Donohue et al., 2006).

In summary, direct priming of naïve $CD8^+$ T cells through TagLuc expression on cancer cells most probably contributed to T cell activation and subsequent cancer cell rejection in the presented model. TCR-HAxRag$^{-/-}$/BALB/c mice used in the described ATT experiment did not express the cognate MHC class I molecule H-2D^b. Consequently, Tag pI could not have been cross-presented by host immune cells, e.g. DCs or macrophages, indicating a direct priming of TCR-I T cells. Furthermore, continuous antigen processing as it is described to be important for direct priming, was ensured starting from the day of TagLuc induction in resting cancer cells. Only rarely transferred non-$CD8^+$ T cells contained in the TCR-I T cell suspension could have led to an unwanted T cell cross-priming. In fact, besides the purified $V\beta7^+$ $CD8^+$ T cells less than 5000 cells have been co-transferred and may have influenced the observed immune responses. However, it is unclear if those cells comprising mainly monocytes, macrophages and NK cells (data not shown) were capable of surviving in a MHC-mismatched, immunodeficient host like a TCR-HAxRag$^{-/-}$/BALB/c mouse. Furthermore, a homing of these non-$CD8^+$ T cells to draining lymph nodes is unlikely to occur and in addition, the capability of these non-$CD8^+$ T cells for antigen uptake and processing remains uncertain. There are only few data existing about persistence of immune cells in the absence of cognate MHC molecule expression and stimulation. Available studies focused mainly on survival of $CD8^+$ T cells but no other cell types such as monocytes or NK cells (Tanchot et al., 1997a; Murali-Krishna et al., 1999).

4.4 Concluding remarks

The aim of this study was to establish and utilize a transplantation model that simulates sporadic tumor formation as it occurs in humans. Application of this model enabled investigation of *de novo* immune responses against neoantigens and answered a central question of immunologists: Is there an interaction of the immune system with emerging cancer cells during sporadic tumor formation and if so, is it protective against tumor growth? The here presented work provides a novel transplantation model that reflects an early phase of sporadic tumorigenesis. Simulating these early phases of cancer development, the model is superior to other mouse cancer models that have been employed in the past for proving the immune surveillance hypothesis. As demonstrated in this study, TagLuc expression by few cancer cells induced a destructive CD8[+] T cell response in immunocompetent CM2 mice under non-acute inflammatory conditions and resulted in cancer cell rejection. For the first time this kind of *de novo* immune response in a model closely mimicking early sporadic tumorigenesis has been established. Hitherto, only few studies reported a *de novo* immune response raised against neoantigens. Different to the presented model wherein the neoantigen was expressed by only few cancer cells, neoantigens used in those studies were expressed by established tumors. Consequently, those findings are not completely comparable to findings provided by the study herein. Moreover, studies describe a spontaneous antibody (Spiotto et al., 2003) or CD4[+] T cell (Flament et al., 2015) response, whereas a spontaneous CD8[+] T cell response was observed in the presented study. The newly induced CD8[+] T cells recognized multiple epitopes of Tag demonstrating that a polyspecific T cell response led to rejection of cancer cells. Further, T cell responses were reliably observed in old mice as well as against cancer cells expressing low amounts of tumor antigen. Applying the novel transplantation model, surveillance of slowly progressing cancer cells by CD8[+] T cells was demonstrated under different conditions. Hence, the hypothesis that the immune system can control new arising cancer cells and eliminate them is supported by the findings of this study. Notably, the cancer-driving oncogene and tumor-specific antigen Tag belongs to an exceptional class of antigens. Its entire amino acid sequence differs from host structures thereby providing multiple antigenic epitopes. This property may increase the probability of the immune system to recognize TagLuc-expressing cancer cells as non-self. Similar antigens are present in some human sporadic cancers, such as colon cancer with a high degree of genetic instability and immune responses against these cancers have been observed in human patients (Reuschenbach et al., 2010; Boissiere-Michot et al., 2014; Maby et al., 2015). But it remains unclear at which time point during cancer development these immune responses were initiated and whether they were ever tumor-destructive. Application of the presented transplantation model demonstrated that destructive immune responses against such a strong antigen like TagLuc can occur already at early phases of tumor development. Furthermore, a potential mechanism of CD8[+] T cell priming in the absence of acute inflammation and classical co-stimulatory molecules expressed by cancer cells was examined in this study. Direct priming was found to take place under different experimental settings. Surprisingly, recognition of TagLuc expressed by cancer cells was independent of CD4[+] T cells and other immune cells that may have cross-presented TagLuc to CD8$^+$ T cells. Contradicting to the major scientific community's belief, direct priming of naïve T cells by nascent cancer cells was found to contribute to tumor immunity. Further efforts are required to elucidate the underlying mechanisms leading to direct priming in the presented model. This includes investigation of involved (co-stimulatory) molecules expressed on cancer and T cells but also localization of T cell priming. Moreover, the presented model provides multiple options for investigation of further issues related to tumor immunology. For example, the relevance of the immune system in controlling cancer cells expressing single tumor-specific epitopes can be determined by introduction of single point mutations – as found in most human cancers. Will expression of such a single epitope in the absence of acute inflammation also lead to tumor-specific immunity?

5 Material and Methods

5.1 Material

5.1.1 Kits

Table 5.1 List of kits

Name	Application	Source
BD OptEIA™ Mouse IFN-γ ELISA	Quantification of IFN-γ in ELISA	BD
DNeasy Blood & Tissue Kit	Cellular DNA extraction	Qiagen
Luciferase Assay System	Cell lysis and luciferase activity measurement	Promega
Mammalian cell lysis kit	Cell lysis and protein extraction	Sigma
Naïve CD8a+ T cell isolation kit	Isolation of naïve CD8+ T cells by MACS	Miltenyi
Naïve CD8a+ T cell isolation kit	Depletion of CD4 T cells by MACS	Miltenyi
Super SignalTM Chemiluminescent Substrate Kit (34080)	Detection of protein-bound antibodies in Western Blot (WB)	Thermo Fisher Scientific

5.1.2 Cell culture media

All cell lines were cultured in Dulbecco's modified eagle medium (Gibco), supplemented with 10 % heat inactivated fetal calf serum (PAN, Biotech) and 50 µg/ml gentamicin (Gibco).

5.1.3 Mouse strains

All mouse strains were housed and bred at the animal facility at Max-Delbrück-Center for Molecular Medicine in the Helmholtz Association, Berlin, Germany.

TCR-I xRag$^{-/-}$ xCD45.1$^{+/+}$ mice were housed at the animal facility of Charité (Campus Benjamin Franklin), Berlin, Germany.

All animal experiments were approved by the Landesamt für Gesundheit und Soziales (LAGeSo), Berlin, and conducted according to institutional and national guidelines and regulations.

Table 5.2 List of mouse strains

Mouse strain	Referred name	Description	Source	Reference
Rag-1$^{-/-}$ and Rag-2$^{-/-}$	Rag$^{-/-}$	deficient for T and B cells	Jackson Laboratory	(Mombaerts et al., 1992)
CAG-rtTA	CM2	Expresses the tetracycline-regulated rtTA2^S-M2 trans-activator under control of a ubiquitously active promoter derived from cyto-megaly virus (CMV)	CM2 mice were generated by pro-nuclei injection into C57BL/6 oocytes	(Anders et al., 2012)
TCR-I	TCR-I	express a transgenic TCR for Tag epitope I	Jackson Laboratory	(Staveley-O'Carroll et al., 2003)
C.129S7(B6)-Rag1^{tm1Mom}/J	Rag$^{-/-}$/BALB/c	deficient for T and B cells MHC class I haplotype: H-2^d	Jackson Laboratory	(Mombaerts et al., 1992)
B10.Cg-H2d Tg(TcraCl4, TcrbCl4)1Shrm/ShrmJ	TCR-HA	express a transgenic TCR for a H-2K^d restricted epitope of hemagglutinin	Jackson Laboratory	(Morgan et al., 1996)
B6.129S7-*Rag1^{tm1Mom}* Tg(TcraT-crb)1100Mjb	Rag$^{-/-}$/OT1	express a transgenic TCR for ovalbumin, deficient for B cells	Taconic	(Hogquist et al., 1994)
B6;B10-*Rag2^{tm1Fwa}* Tg(TcrLCMV)327Sdz	P14xRag$^{-/-}$	Express a transgenic TCR for LCMV gp33, deficient for B cells	Taconic	(Pircher et al., 1989)
B6.SJL-*Ptprc^a* Pepc^b/BoyJ	CD45.1$^{+/+}$	congenic strain expressing CD45.1 (Ly5.1)	Jackson Laboratory	(Shen et al., 1985)
C57BL/6-Tyr^{c-Brd}	albino B6	spontaneous mutation (transversion) in tyrosinase gene leads to albinism	Jackson Laboratory	(Liu et al., 1998)

5.1.4 Cell lines

Table 5.3 List of cell lines Displayed is each cell line and its origin used for experiments in the presented study. n.d. = not determined

Name	Type	Description	Species	Reference
TC200.09	n.d.	tumor cell line derived from sporadic tumor of a $TRE^{loxP}stop^{loxP}TagLuc$ xCAG-rtTA (TC) transgenic mouse	$TRE^{loxP}stop^{loxP}Tag$-Luc xCAG-rtTA mouse (C57Bl/6)	(Anders et al., 2011)
Clone 4	n.d.	clonal cancer cell line derived from TC200.09	$TRE^{loxP}stop^{loxP}Tag$-Luc xCAG-rtTA mouse (C57Bl/6)	unpublished
MCA-205	fibrosarcoma	3-methylcholanthrene (MCA) induced	C57BL/6 (B6) mouse	(Barth et al., 1990)
Tet-TagLuc	fibroblastic cells	Tag expressing cancer cell line derived from fibroblasts of a transgenic mouse	$TRE^{loxP}stop^{loxP}Tag$-Luc mouse (B6)	(Anders et al., 2011)
TTC #3055	spindle cell tumor	TagLuc expressing cancer cell line isolated from a transgenic mouse	$TRE^{loxP}stop^{loxP}Tag$-Luc xCAG-rtTA xTyrCre mouse	(Anders et al., 2017)
CY-15	histiocytoma	7,12-dimethylbenz(a)anthracene (DMBA) / 2-O-tetradecanoylphorbol-13-acetate (TPA) induced	BALB/c IFNγ$^{-/-}$ mouse	(Kammertoens et al., 2005)
B16.F10	melanoma	tumor cell line isolated from a C57Bl/6 mouse	B6 mouse	(Fidler, 1975)

5.1.5 Adenovirus

A recombinant and replication deficient adenovirus encoding a CMV promoter-driven *nls* Cre gene (Willimsky and Blankenstein, 2005) was used.

5.1.6 Oligonucleotides for PCR

Table 5.4 List of oligonucleotides used for PCR

Primer name	Sequence	Application	Primer flanked sequence	Amplification product length [bp]
seCM2 asCM2	5' GCCTGACGACAAGGA AACTC 3' 5' AGCCTTGCTGACACAGGAAC 3'	Genotyping	rtTA	248
seTRE1 asCAT	5'GCGTGTACGGTGGGAGGCCTA 3' 5' CGGATGAGCATTCATCAGGCGGG 3'	Recombination PCR	TRE^{loxP}stop^{loxP}Tag-Luc	439 / none*
seTRE2 asTag	5' CGAGGTAGGCGTGTACGGTGG 3' 5' GCAAATTTAAAGCGCTGATGATCC 3'	Recombination PCR	TRE^{loxP}stop^{loxP}Tag-Luc	1925 / 283*
seTRE1 asCAT asTag	5'GCGTGTACGGTGGGAGGCCTA 3' 5' CGGATGAGCATTCATCAGGCGGG 3' 5' GCAAATTTAAAGCGCTGATGATCC 3'	Recombination PCR	TRE^{loxP}stop^{loxP}Tag-Luc	439 / 275*

* product amplified after deletion of stop cassette chloramphenicol acetyltransferase (CAT)

5.1.7 Antibodies and tetramers

Table 5.5 List of antibodies and tetramers

Specificity	Conjugate	Clone	Isotype	Host	Application	Source
mouse β-actin	-	polyclonal	IgG	rabbit	WB	abcam
mouse β-actin	HRP	AC-15	IgG1	mouse	WB	Sigma
SV40 T antigen	-	Pab416	IgG2α	mouse	WB	Calbiochem
mouse p16	-	polyclonal	IgG	rabbit	WB	Santa Cruz
mouse p21	-	polyclonal	IgG	rabbit	WB	Santa Cruz
mouse histone H3 (tri me-thyl K9)	-	polyclonal	IgG	rabbit	WB	abcam
rabbit IgG	HRP	polyclonal	IgG	goat	WB	SouthernBiotech
mouse IgG	HRP	polyclonal	IgG	goat	WB	SouthernBiotech
goat IgG	HRP	polyclonal	IgG	rabbit	WB	SouthernBiotech
BrdU	APC	Bu20a	IgG1, κ	mouse	FC	Biolegend
mouse CD3ε	APC or FITC	145-2C11	IgG	Armenian hamster	FC	Biolegend
mouse CD4	APC	RM4-5	IgG2α, κ	rat	FC	Biolegend

Specificity	Conjugate	Clone	Isotype	Host	Application	Source
mouse CD8a	APC or BV421	53–6.7	IgG2α, κ	rat	FC	Biolegend
mouse Vβ7 TCR	FITC	TR310	IgG2b, κ	rat	FC	Biolegend
mouse H-2D^b/H-2K^b	biotin	28-8-6	IgG2α, κ	mouse	FC	Biolegend
biotin	PE	1D4-C5	IgG2α, κ	mouse	FC	Biolegend
mouse CD45.1	APC	A20	IgG2α, κ	mouse	FC	Biolegend
mouse CD80	PE	16-10A1	IgG	Armenian hamster	FC	Biolegend
mouse CD86	PE	GL-1	IgG2α, κ	rat	FC	Biolegend
mouse CD54	FITC	3E2	IgG1, κ	Armenian hamster	FC	BD
mouse CD44	APC	MEL14	IgG2α, κ	rat	FC	Biolegend
mouse CD62L	PE	IM7	IgG2b, κ	rat	FC	Biolegend
Armenian hamster IgG (isotype control)	PE	HTK888	-	-	FC	Biolegend
Armenian hamster IgG1, κ (isotype control)	FITC	A19-3	-	-	FC	BD
mouse IgG2α, κ (isotype control)	PE	G155-178	-	-	FC	BD
rat IgG2α, κ (isotype control)	PE	R35-95	-	-	FC	BD
H-2D^b/SAINNYAQKL (Tag peptide I) tetramer	PE	-	-	-	FC	Biozol/MBL
H-2K^b/ VVYDFLKL (Tag peptide IV) tetramer	PE	-	-	-	FC	Biozol/MBL

Abbreviations: APC, allophycocyanin; BV, brilliant violet; FC, flow cytometry; FITC, fluorescein isothiocyanate; HRP, horse radish peroxidase; PE, phycoerythrin; WB, western blot.

5.2   Methods

5.2.1   Selection of cancer cell lines with conditional TagLuc expression

To establish a cancer cell line that allows proliferation and oncogene/antigen regulation *in vivo* and subsequently, study of spontaneous T cell responses, we selected TC200.09. The gastric cancer cell line TC200.09 was isolated from a double transgenic TRE^{loxP}stop^{loxP}Tag-Luc x CAG-rtTA mouse. This sporadic tumor occurred 411 d after dox treatment, which has led to somatic mutations or epigenetic events. The cell line has been passaged once in a Rag$^{-/-}$ mouse and a new cell line (TC200.09) was established from the resulting tumor (Anders et al., 2011). Subsequently, the loxP-flanked stop cassette was deleted by infecting the cells with a Cre recombinase -encoding adenovirus (AdCre). Cells were seeded in 24-well plate at a confluency of $\approx$ 90 % and 4 µl of AdCre diluted in 200 µl DMEM were added to cells that were then incubated 90 minutes (min) at 32 °C. After incubation, medium volume was increased to 1 ml followed by a medium exchange after additional 16 h of incubation. The resulting bulk culture of TC200.09 cells did not harbor the stop cassette and underwent a cloning by limiting dilution. To this end, 0,3 cells/well were seeded in four 96-well plates and each well was checked every 2 d for growth of single cell colonies. Single cell clones were expanded and subsequently, tested for successful recombination of stop cassette by PCR. Single cell clone 4F5, later always referred to as 'clone 4', was selected and used for experiments.

The TTC #3055 cancer cell line was isolated from a sporadic tumor occurring 435 d after dox treatment in a triple transgenic mouse (TRE^{loxP}stop^{loxP}TagLuc x CAG-rtTA x TyrCre). The tumor grew craniofacial in proximity to the snout and is of spindle cell origin. Furthermore, the cancer cells derived from that tumor showed no tyrosinase promoter activity and thus, Cre recombinase is also not expressed (Anders et al., 2017).

5.2.2   Cancer cell transplantation

Cancer cells were seeded in different sized cell culture flasks (TPP) at a confluency of 70 to 90 %. For inactivation of TagLuc expression, cancer cells were cultured in the absence of dox for 14 d. Then, cells were harvested by adding trypsin (Gibco) for 5 min, washed once with phosphate buffered saline (PBS) and resuspended in PBS mixed with BD Matrigel^{TM} (Becton Dickinson, BD) to a final concentration of 10 mg/ml. Cells were stored on ice until inoculation into mice. 1×10^3 to 1×10^5 cancer cells were inoculated subcutaneously (s.c.) by using a needle sized of 27 Gauges (B. Braun).

Tumor volumes were measured along three orthogonal axes (x, y and z) by a caliper and calculated according to the formula volume = $(x \ast y \ast z)/2$

5.2.3   Doxycycline treatment

Mice received dox via drinking water. Therefore, water containing 200 µg/ml dox (Sigma) and 5 % sucrose (Sigma) were provided in light-protected bottles and exchanged twice a week. Cells were supplied with 1 µg/ml dox in the medium which was changed every 2 to 3 d.

5.2.4 Luciferase activity assay

Cells cultured in 6-well plates were harvested as followed: medium was removed, cells were washed once with PBS and 500 µl of Reporter lysis buffer (Promega) was added for 1 to 2 min. Cell harvest was supported by using a cell scraper. Cell suspension was transferred to 1,5 ml Eppendorf shock-frozen with liquid nitrogen for 2 min. After thawing on ice, cell lysate was subjected to 10-min centrifugation at 12.000 rpm with a table top centrifuge (Eppendorf) at 4 °C, supernatant containing proteins was collected and stored at -80 °C. 10 µl of proteins were mixed with Luciferase assay buffer (Promega) and Luciferase substrate buffer (Promega), respectively, and assayed for Fluc activity using a Mithras LB 940 luminometer (Berthold Technologies). Protein concentration was determined by Bradford Assay (Roti®Quant) and relative light unit (RLU) measured in the assay was calculated according to total µg protein.

5.2.5 *In vitro* T cell antigen recognition assay

$1x10^5$ cancer cells were co-cultured with $1x10^6$ TCR-I T cells in RPMI medium supplemented with 10 % FCS, 10 mM HEPES and 50 µM β-mercaptoethanol. Previously, TCR-I T cells were isolated from spleen of a SV40 TCR I transgenic mouse. Briefly, spleen was cut into small pieces, smashed through a 40 µm cell strainer and spun down at 1200 rpm for 5 min. Erythrocytes were lysed by adding ACK lysis buffer (Gibco) for 3 min, followed by 3 times of washing with PBS. TCR-I T cells were labelled with 2 µM CellTrace™ CFSE (Life technologies). After 5 d of co-culture, T cells were collected and stained with mouse anti-CD3 and mouse anti-CD8 antibodies. CFSE dilution as parameter for proliferation was detected by flow cytometry.

5.2.6 *In vivo* T cell proliferation assay

For the *in vivo* T cell proliferation assay, splenocytes from a TCR-I xRag$^{-/-}$ xCD45.1$^{+/+}$ mouse were isolated and subsequently proceeded as described before. $1x10^5$ CFSE-labelled T cells diluted in 100 µl PBS were injected intravenously into recipient mice. In addition, $1x10^5$ cancer cells ('on dox' or 'off dox') solved in 100 µl PBS containing 10 mg/ml BD Matrigel™ were inoculated s.c. into flank. Mice inoculated with cancer cells 'on dox' received dox to sustain TagLuc expression during the experiment. After 5 d, draining and non-draining inguinal lymph nodes were isolated. Lymph nodes were smashed through a 40 µm cell strainer and washed once with PBS. After 5 min of centrifugation at 1200 rpm, cells were stained with mouse anti-CD45.1 and mouse anti-CD8 antibodies, and CFSE dilution was detected by flow cytometry.

5.2.7 Flow cytometry

Expression of surface antigens was detected by incubation of cells (up to $1x10^6$) with 0.2 to 0.5 µg specific monoclonal antibodies in 50 µl PBS for 15 to 30 min at 4 °C. Cells were washed once with PBS and resolved in 200 µl PBS before analysis using a FACS Canto II device (BD). Data was analyzed with FlowJo software (Treestar, Ashland, Oregon, USA). Detection of functional TCR expression on peripheral blood T cells was achieved by incubation with MHC/peptide tetramers for 15 min at room temperature (RT).

Erythrocyte lysis in peripheral blood samples was performed with BD lysing solution prior to FACS measurement. BD lysing solution was added for 8 to 10 min followed by one wash with PBS.

5.2.8 Bioluminescent imaging

In vivo bioluminescent imaging (BLI) was performed using a Xenogen IVIS 200 device (Caliper Life Sciences, Waltham, Massachusetts, USA). Mice were anesthetized by isoflurane inhalation and injected intravenously (i.v.) with 3 mg D-Luciferin (Biosynth) dissolved in PBS (30 mg/ml). Mice were placed immediately after substrate injection in a light tight chamber and whole body and luminescent image photographs were acquired. Acquisition conditions were set up dependent on signal strength and varied between 1 second (s) and 60 s exposure time. The luminescence image is displayed as a false-color image: red color represents a high light signal and purple color a lower light signal. Living image software (version 2.6, Caliper Life Sciences) was used to analyze BL data by overlay of both images and quantification of BL signal.

5.2.9 Immunoblotting

For determination of TagLuc expression in cancer cells, proteins were isolated from cultured cells (Mammalian Cell Lysis Kit, Sigma-Aldrich) and used in a standard Western blot. 35 µg protein were separated on a NuPage™ 4-12 % Bis-Tris SDS gel (Invitrogen) and blotted on a nitrocellulose membrane (GE Healthcare) utilizing a XCell II blot module (Invitrogen). The membrane was incubated in blocking buffer (TRIS-Base buffered saline (TBS) supplemented with 0.05 % Tween-20 and 5 % milk powder) for 1 h followed by 3 times of washing for 10 min with washing buffer (TBS supplemented with 0.05 % Tween-20). Primary antibody (2.5 µg/ml SV40-Tag IgG2α) was diluted in blocking buffer and applied to membrane for 16 h at 4 °C upon agitation. After 3 times of washing for 10 min with washing buffer, the membrane was incubated with secondary antibody (0.1 µg/ml rat anti-mouse IgG2α labelled with horseradish peroxidase (HRP)) for 1 h at RT. After 5 times of washing with washing buffer, chemiluminescence signal was visualized using the Super Signal™ Chemiluminescent Substrate Kit (Thermo Fisher) and the LUMI-F1 imaging workstation (Roche). Additionally, the membrane was incubated with monoclonal mouse anti-β actin antibody labelled with HRP to relate protein expression to total protein load.

5.2.10 BrdU incorporation assay

Replication dependent proliferative activity of cancer cells was assayed by incorporation of 5-bromo-2'-deoxyuridine (BrdU) into DNA. Therefore, cells were pulsed with 10 µM BrdU (Sigma) dissolved in PBS for 60 min. After BrdU pulse, cells were washed once with PBS and harvested. Permeabilization was accomplished by resuspension of cells in ice-cold 70 %

ethanol mixed with PBS and storage for at least 2 h at -20 °C. Subsequently, preparation of cells for staining with monoclonal anti-BrdU antibody was performed as followed: Cells were washed once with PBS, incubated with 2 ml 2N HCl/0.5 % Triton X-100 for 30 min, spun down and incubated with 2 ml 0.1 M sodium tetraborate (Sigma) for 10 min. After 2 times of washing with PBS, cells were incubated with anti-BrdU antibody (Biolegend) diluted in PBS supplemented with 0.5 % Tween-20 and 1 % BSA for 30 min at RT. Subsequently, cells were incubated with 20 μg/ml propidium iodide (PI, solved in PBS containing 0.5 % Tween-20, 1 % BSA and 10 μg/ml RNase A (Qiagen)) for 30 min at RT. Cells in different cell cycle phases were determined in a FACS by analysis of BrdU incorporation in viable (PI positive) cells.

5.2.11 INF-γ ELISA

IFN-γ production by TCR-I T cells was measured by enzyme-linked immunosorbent assay (ELISA). Undiluted supernatants from a 5-d co-culture of naïve TCR-I T cells with cancer cells were analyzed by utilizing the BD OptEIA Mouse IFN-γ ELISA set (Becton Dickinson, BD). ELISA was performed according to the manufacturer's instructions.

5.2.12 DNA amplification and detection of recombination

DNA for detection of stop cassette deletion in cancer cells was isolated using the DNeasy Blood & Tissue Kit (Qiagen). For genotyping, DNA was isolated from tail biopsies by boiling the tail piece in 0.05 M NaOH at 95 °C for 1 h. The reaction was stopped by adding 50 μl of 1 M Tris/10 mM EDTA solution. Polymerase chain reaction (PCR) was carried out by preparing the following reaction mixture and using the following PCR protocol:

Table 5.6 List of ingredients for genotyping PCR

Reagent	Volume [μl]	Final concentration
DNA template (≤ 1 μg)	1	
dNTPS (10 mM each)	0.2	5 μM
MgCl₂ (25 mM)	1	25 μM
Forward primer (10 mM)	0.5	5 μM
Reverse primer (10 mM)	0.5	5 μM
Taq polymerase (5U/μl)	0.1	0.5 μM
ddH₂O	ad 10	

Table 5.7 List of steps and respective settings for genotyping PCR

Step	Time	Temperature	Number of cycles
Polymerase activation	5 min	95°C	
DNA denaturation	30 s	95°C	
Primer annealing	30 s	60°C	x 30
Primer extension	60 s	72°C	
Final elongation	10 min	72°C	

The amplification products were separated on a 1 % agarose gel supplemented with ethidium bromide (0.4 µg/ml) together with size marker (1 kb ladder, Fermentas). DNA bands were visualized by using a LUMI-F1 imaging workstation (Roche).

5.2.13 *In vitro* direct priming assay

Naïve CD8$^+$ T cells were isolated from spleen of a TCR-I transgenic mouse by magnetic-activated cell sorting (MACS) using the Naïve CD8a$^+$ T cell isolation kit (Miltenyi). Briefly, spleen was cut into small pieces, smashed through a 40 µm cell strainer and spun down at 1200 rpm for 5 min. Erythrocytes were lysed by adding ACK lysis buffer (Gibco) for 3 min, followed by 2 times of washing with PBS. After erythrocyte lysis with ACK lysis buffer, cells were taken up in MACS buffer (PBS, 0.5 % FCS, 2 mM EDTA) according to the manufacturer's protocol. After addition of an antibody cocktail, containing biotin-conjugated antibodies against CD45R, CD4, CD11b, CD11c, CD19, CD44, CD49b, CD105, Ter-119, MHC II, and anti-TCRγ/δ, the cells were incubated for 10 min at 4 °C and anti-biotin MicroBeads (Miltenyi) were added for subsequent depletion of the cells. After 15 min incubation cells were washed with MACS buffer, a LS MACS column (Miltenyi) was placed into a MACS separator (Milteny) and equilibrated with 3 ml MACS buffer. The cells resuspended in MACS buffer, were applied to column and the column was washed 3 times with MACS buffer. The naïve CD8$^+$ T cell containing effluent was collected and cells were washed with PBS and counted. An aliquot was stained with monoclonal mouse anti-Vβ7, anti-CD8a. anti-CD44 and anti-CD62L antibody and subjected to flow cytometry analysis to confirm cell purity.

5×10^5 negative selected naïve TCR-I T cells were cultured together with 5×10^4 cancer cells for 3 d. If required, dox was added to culture. 1 µM Tag pI peptide was exogenously loaded on cancer cells by incubating cells with the peptide for 2 h, followed by 2 times of washing with PBS. After 3 d of co-culture, T cells were collected, stained with monoclonal mouse anti-CD3, anti-CD8 and anti-CD69 antibody and analyzed by flow cytometry.

5.2.14 *In vivo* direct priming assay

Recipient mice were inoculated with 1×10^4 clone 4 cancer cells 'off dox' (in 100 µl PBS containing 10 mg/ml BD Matrigel™). Dox was administered to the mice via drinking water 4 weeks post cancer cell inoculation. 5 d after dox administration, 1×10^5 naïve MACS-sorted TCR-I T cells in 100 µl PBS were injected intravenously. Naïve TCR-I T cells were isolated as followed: splenocytes of 3 TCR-I transgenic mouse were isolated as described before, and pooled prior MACS sort of naïve T cells with the Naïve CD8a$^+$ T cell isolation kit (Miltenyi). MACS sort was performed as described in the section before. An aliquot of the effluent containing the naïve CD8$^+$ T cells was stained with monoclonal mouse anti-Vβ7, anti-CD8a, anti-CD44 and anti CD62L antibody and subjected to flow cytometry analysis to confirm cell purity.

5.2.15 CD4$^+$ T cell depletion experiment

P14xRag$^{-/-}$ mice were inoculated with 1×10^4 clone 4 cancer cells 'off dox' (in 100 µl PBS containing 10 mg/ml BD Matrigel™) and dox was administered to the mice via drinking water 2 weeks post cell inoculation. At the time of dox administration, splenocytes isolated from naïve CM2 mice and containing 1×10^6 CD8$^+$ T cells (in 100 µl PBS) were adoptively transferred through intravenous injection. Spleens from 4 naïve CM2 mice were isolated, cut in half, pooled and processed either for CD4$^+$ T cell-depletion by MACS or left untreated. Splenocyte suspension from pooled spleen halves was depleted of CD4$^+$ T cells by use of CD4 (L3T4) MicroBeads (Miltenyi) and MACS according to the manufacturer's protocol. An aliquot of the effluent was stained with monoclonal mouse anti-CD3, anti-CD4 and anti-CD8 antibodies for analysis by flow cytometry to confirm depletion of CD4$^+$ T cells and calculate the number of CD8$^+$ T cells contained within.

5.3 Suppliers

Abcam (Cambridge, UK)

B. Braun (Melsungen, Germany)

BD Biosciences (Franklin Lakes, New Jersey, USA)

Berthold Technologies (Bad Wildbad, Germany)

Biolegend (San Diego, California, USA)

Biosynth (Staat, Switzerland)

Biozol Diagnostica (Eching, Germany)

Caliper Life Sciences (Waltham, Massachusetts, USA)

Fermentas (Waltham, Massachusetts, USA)

GE Healthcare (Buckinghamshire, UK)

Gibco (Karlsruhe, Germany)

Invitrogen (Karlsruhe, Germany)

Life Technologies (Carlsbad, California, USA)

Miltenyi Biotec (Bergisch Gladbach, Germany)

PAN Biotech (Aidenbach, Germany)

Promega (Madison, Wisconsin, USA)

Qiagen (Hilden, Germany)

Roche (Basel, Schweiz)

Sigma-Aldrich (St. Louis, Missouri, USA)

SouthernBiotech (Birmingham, Alabama, USA)

Thermo Fisher Scientific (Waltham, Massachusetts, USA)

Tree Star (Ashland, Oregon, USA)

6 Bibliography

Ahuja, D., Saenz-Robles, M. T., and Pipas, J. M. (2005). SV40 large T antigen targets multiple cellular pathways to elicit cellular transformation. Oncogene *24*, 7729-7745.

Alexandrov, L. B., Nik-Zainal, S., Wedge, D. C., Aparicio, S. A., Behjati, S., Biankin, A. V., Bignell, G. R., Bolli, N., Borg, A., Borresen-Dale, A. L., *et al.* (2013). Signatures of mutational processes in human cancer. Nature *500*, 415-421.

Anders, K., Buschow, C., Charo, J., and Blankenstein, T. (2012). Depot formation of doxycycline impairs Tet-regulated gene expression in vivo. Transgenic Res *21*, 1099-1107.

Anders, K., Buschow, C., Herrmann, A., Milojkovic, A., Loddenkemper, C., Kammertoens, T., Daniel, P., Yu, H., Charo, J., and Blankenstein, T. (2011). Oncogene-targeting T cells reject large tumors while oncogene inactivation selects escape variants in mouse models of cancer. Cancer Cell *20*, 755-767.

Anders, K., Kershaw, O., Larue, L., Gruber, A. D., and Blankenstein, T. (2017). The immune system prevents recurrence of transplanted but not autochthonous antigenic tumors after oncogene inactivation therapy. Int J Cancer *141*, 2551-2561.

Anderson, M. S., and Su, M. A. (2011). Aire and T cell development. Curr Opin Immunol *23*, 198-206.

Antony, P. A., Piccirillo, C. A., Akpinarli, A., Finkelstein, S. E., Speiss, P. J., Surman, D. R., Palmer, D. C., Chan, C. C., Klebanoff, C. A., Overwijk, W. W., *et al.* (2005). CD8+ T cell immunity against a tumor/self-antigen is augmented by CD4+ T helper cells and hindered by naturally occurring T regulatory cells. J Immunol *174*, 2591-2601.

Armitage, P., and Doll, R. (1954). The age distribution of cancer and a multi-stage theory of carcinogenesis. Br J Cancer *8*, 1-12.

Bai, X. F., Gao, J. X., Liu, J., Wen, J., Zheng, P., and Liu, Y. (2001). On the site and mode of antigen presentation for the initiation of clonal expansion of CD8 T cells specific for a natural tumor antigen. Cancer Res *61*, 6860-6867.

Bakker, A. B., Schreurs, M. W., de Boer, A. J., Kawakami, Y., Rosenberg, S. A., Adema, G. J., and Figdor, C. G. (1994). Melanocyte lineage-specific antigen gp100 is recognized by melanoma-derived tumor-infiltrating lymphocytes. J Exp Med *179*, 1005-1009.

Barth, R. J., Jr., Bock, S. N., Mule, J. J., and Rosenberg, S. A. (1990). Unique murine tumor-associated antigens identified by tumor infiltrating lymphocytes. J Immunol *144*, 1531-1537.

Basingab, F. S., Ahmadi, M., and Morgan, D. J. (2016). IFNgamma-Dependent Interactions between ICAM-1 and LFA-1 Counteract Prostaglandin E2-Mediated Inhibition of Antitumor CTL Responses. Cancer Immunol Res *4*, 400-411.

Beheshti, A., Benzekry, S., McDonald, J. T., Ma, L., Peluso, M., Hahnfeldt, P., and Hlatky, L. (2015). Host age is a systemic regulator of gene expression impacting cancer progression. Cancer Res *75*, 1134-1143.

Bellovin, D. I., Das, B., and Felsher, D. W. (2013). Tumor dormancy, oncogene addiction, cellular senescence, and self-renewal programs. Adv Exp Med Biol *734*, 91-107.

Bennett, C. L., and Chakraverty, R. (2012). Dendritic cells in tissues: in situ stimulation of immunity and immunopathology. Trends Immunol *33*, 8-13.

Bevan, M. J. (1976). Cross-priming for a secondary cytotoxic response to minor H antigens with H-2 congenic cells which do not cross-react in the cytotoxic assay. Journal of Experimental Medicine *143*, 1283-1288.

Bikel, I., Montano, X., Agha, M. E., Brown, M., McCormack, M., Boltax, J., and Livingston, D. M. (1987). SV40 small t antigen enhances the transformation activity of limiting concentrations of SV40 large T antigen. Cell *48*, 321-330.

Bissell, M. J., and Radisky, D. (2001). Putting tumours in context. Nat Rev Cancer *1*, 46-54.

Blankenstein, T., Coulie, P. G., Gilboa, E., and Jaffee, E. M. (2012). The determinants of tumour immunogenicity. Nat Rev Cancer *12*, 307-313.

Blankenstein, T., and Qin, Z. (2003). Chemical carcinogens as foreign bodies and some pitfalls regarding cancer immune surveillance. Adv Cancer Res *90*, 179-207.

Boissiere-Michot, F., Lazennec, G., Frugier, H., Jarlier, M., Roca, L., Duffour, J., Du Paty, E., Laune, D., Blanchard, F., Le Pessot, F., *et al.* (2014). Characterization of an adaptive immune response in microsatellite-instable colorectal cancer. Oncoimmunology *3*, e29256.

Boon, T., and van der Bruggen, P. (1996). Human tumor antigens recognized by T lymphocytes. J Exp Med *183*, 725-729.

Boonman, Z. F., van Mierlo, G. J., Fransen, M. F., Franken, K. L., Offringa, R., Melief, C. J., Jager, M. J., and Toes, R. E. (2004). Intraocular tumor antigen drains specifically to submandibular lymph nodes, resulting in an abortive cytotoxic T cell reaction. J Immunol *172*, 1567-1574.

Bos, R., and Sherman, L. A. (2010). CD4+ T-cell help in the tumor milieu is required for recruitment and cytolytic function of CD8+ T lymphocytes. Cancer Res *70*, 8368-8377.

Bretscher, P., and Cohn, M. (1970). A theory of self-nonself discrimination. Science *169*, 1042-1049.

Briesemeister, D., Friese, C., Isern, C. C., Dietz, E., Blankenstein, T., Thoene-Reineke, C., and Kammertoens, T. (2012). Differences in serum cytokine levels between wild type mice and mice with a targeted mutation suggests necessity of using control littermates. Cytokine *60*, 626-633.

Bringold, F., and Serrano, M. (2000). Tumor suppressors and oncogenes in cellular senescence. Exp Gerontol *35*, 317-329.

Brinster, R. L., Chen, H. Y., Messing, A., van Dyke, T., Levine, A. J., and Palmiter, R. D. (1984). Transgenic mice harboring SV40 T-antigen genes develop characteristic brain tumors. Cell *37*, 367-379.

Brodsky, J. L., and Pipas, J. M. (1998). Polyomavirus T antigens: molecular chaperones for multiprotein complexes. Journal of virology *72*, 5329-5334.

Burnet, F. M. (1961). Immunological recognition of self. Science *133*, 307-311.

Burnet, M. (1957). Cancer; a biological approach. I. The processes of control. Br Med J *1*, 779-786.

Burstein, N. A., and Law, L. W. (1971). Neonatal thymectomy and non-viral mammary tumours in mice. Nature *231*, 450-452.

Buschow, C., Charo, J., Anders, K., Loddenkemper, C., Jukica, A., Alsamah, W., Perez, C., Willimsky, G., and Blankenstein, T. (2010). In vivo imaging of an inducible oncogenic tumor antigen visualizes tumor progression and predicts CTL tolerance. J Immunol *184*, 2930-2938.

Call, K. M., Glaser, T., Ito, C. Y., Buckler, A. J., Pelletier, J., Haber, D. A., Rose, E. A., Kral, A., Yeger, H., Lewis, W. H., and et al. (1990). Isolation and characterization of a zinc finger polypeptide gene at the human chromosome 11 Wilms' tumor locus. Cell *60*, 509-520.

Carbone, M., Pass, H. I., Miele, L., and Bocchetta, M. (2003). New developments about the association of SV40 with human mesothelioma. Oncogene *22*, 5173-5180.

Chen, L., Linsley, P. S., and Hellstrom, K. E. (1993). Costimulation of T cells for tumor immunity. Immunol Today *14*, 483-486.

Chen, W., Masterman, K. A., Basta, S., Haeryfar, S. M., Dimopoulos, N., Knowles, B., Bennink, J. R., and Yewdell, J. W. (2004). Cross-priming of CD8+ T cells by viral and tumor antigens is a robust phenomenon. Eur J Immunol *34*, 194-199.

Church, S. E., Jensen, S. M., Antony, P. A., Restifo, N. P., and Fox, B. A. (2014). Tumor-specific CD4+ T cells maintain effector and memory tumor-specific CD8+ T cells. Eur J Immunol *44*, 69-79.

Clemente, C. G., Mihm, M. C., Jr., Bufalino, R., Zurrida, S., Collini, P., and Cascinelli, N. (1996). Prognostic value of tumor infiltrating lymphocytes in the vertical growth phase of primary cutaneous melanoma. Cancer *77*, 1303-1310.

Connolly, D. C., Bao, R., Nikitin, A. Y., Stephens, K. C., Poole, T. W., Hua, X., Harris, S. S., Vanderhyden, B. C., and Hamilton, T. C. (2003). Female mice chimeric for expression of the simian virus 40 TAg under control of the MISIIR promoter develop epithelial ovarian cancer. Cancer research *63*, 1389-1397.

Coppe, J. P., Patil, C. K., Rodier, F., Sun, Y., Munoz, D. P., Goldstein, J., Nelson, P. S., Desprez, P. Y., and Campisi, J. (2008). Senescence-associated secretory phenotypes reveal cell-nonautonomous functions of oncogenic RAS and the p53 tumor suppressor. PLoS Biol *6*, 2853-2868.

Corthay, A., Skovseth, D. K., Lundin, K. U., Rosjo, E., Omholt, H., Hofgaard, P. O., Haraldsen, G., and Bogen, B. (2005). Primary antitumor immune response mediated by CD4+ T cells. Immunity *22*, 371-383.

Coulie, P. G., Lehmann, F., Lethe, B., Herman, J., Lurquin, C., Andrawiss, M., and Boon, T. (1995). A mutated intron sequence codes for an antigenic peptide recognized by cytolytic T lymphocytes on a human melanoma. Proc Natl Acad Sci U S A *92*, 7976-7980.

Coussens, L., Yang-Feng, T. L., Liao, Y. C., Chen, E., Gray, A., McGrath, J., Seeburg, P. H., Libermann, T. A., Schlessinger, J., Francke, U., and et al. (1985). Tyrosine kinase receptor with extensive homology to EGF receptor shares chromosomal location with neu oncogene. Science *230*, 1132-1139.

Dash, B. C., and El-Deiry, W. S. (2005). Phosphorylation of p21 in G2/M promotes cyclin B-Cdc2 kinase activity. Molecular and cellular biology *25*, 3364-3387.

de Wet, J. R., Wood, K. V., Helinski, D. R., and DeLuca, M. (1985). Cloning of firefly luciferase cDNA and the expression of active luciferase in Escherichia coli. Proc Natl Acad Sci U S A *82*, 7870-7873.

DeCaprio, J. A., and Garcea, R. L. (2013). A cornucopia of human polyomaviruses. Nat Rev Microbiol *11*, 264-276.

DeCaprio, J. A., Ludlow, J. W., Figge, J., Shew, J. Y., Huang, C. M., Lee, W. H., Marsilio, E., Paucha, E., and Livingston, D. M. (1988). SV40 large tumor antigen forms a specific complex with the product of the retinoblastoma susceptibility gene. Cell *54*, 275-283.

Derhovanessian, E., Solana, R., Larbi, A., and Pawelec, G. (2008). Immunity, ageing and cancer. Immun Ageing *5*, 11.

Dolcetti, R., Viel, A., Doglioni, C., Russo, A., Guidoboni, M., Capozzi, E., Vecchiato, N., Macri, E., Fornasarig, M., and Boiocchi, M. (1999). High prevalence of activated intraepithelial cytotoxic T lymphocytes and increased neoplastic cell apoptosis in colorectal carcinomas with microsatellite instability. Am J Pathol *154*, 1805-1813.

Donohue, K. B., Grant, J. M., Tewalt, E. F., Palmer, D. C., Theoret, M. R., Restifo, N. P., and Norbury, C. C. (2006). Cross-priming utilizes antigen not available to the direct presentation pathway. Immunology *119*, 63-73.

Dubois, N., Bennoun, M., Allemand, I., Molina, T., Grimber, G., Daudet-Monsac, M., Abelanet, R., and Briand, P. (1991). Time-course development of differentiated hepatocarcinoma and lung metastasis in transgenic mice. Journal of hepatology *13*, 227-239.

Dudley, M. E., Wunderlich, J. R., Yang, J. C., Hwu, P., Schwartzentruber, D. J., Topalian, S. L., Sherry, R. M., Marincola, F. M., Leitman, S. F., and Seipp, C. A. (2002). A phase I study of nonmyeloablative chemotherapy and adoptive transfer of autologous tumor antigen-specific T lymphocytes in patients with metastatic melanoma. Journal of immunotherapy (Hagerstown, Md: 1997) *25*, 243.

Dunn, G. P., Bruce, A. T., Ikeda, H., Old, L. J., and Schreiber, R. D. (2002). Cancer immunoediting: from immunosurveillance to tumor escape. Nat Immunol *3*, 991-998.

Dunn, G. P., Old, L. J., and Schreiber, R. D. (2004). The immunobiology of cancer immunosurveillance and immunoediting. Immunity *21*, 137-148.

DuPage, M., Cheung, A. F., Mazumdar, C., Winslow, M. M., Bronson, R., Schmidt, L. M., Crowley, D., Chen, J., and Jacks, T. (2011). Endogenous T cell responses to antigens expressed in lung adenocarcinomas delay malignant tumor progression. Cancer Cell *19*, 72-85.

Eddy, B. E., Borman, G. S., Grubbs, G. E., and Young, R. D. (1962). Identification of the oncogenic substance in rhesus monkey kidney cell cultures as simian virus 40. Virology *17*, 65-75.

Edinger, M., Sweeney, T. J., Tucker, A. A., Olomu, A. B., Negrin, R. S., and Contag, C. H. (1999). Noninvasive assessment of tumor cell proliferation in animal models. Neoplasia *1*, 303-310.

Ehrlich, P. (1909). Ueber den jetzigen Stand der Karzinomforschung. Ned Tijdschr Geneeskd, 8.

Ewald, J. A., Desotelle, J. A., Wilding, G., and Jarrard, D. F. (2010). Therapy-induced senescence in cancer. J Natl Cancer Inst *102*, 1536-1546.

Fan, D. N., and Schmitt, C. A. (2017). Detecting Markers of Therapy-Induced Senescence in Cancer Cells. Methods Mol Biol *1534*, 41-52.

Farge, D. (1993). Kaposi's sarcoma in organ transplant recipients. The Collaborative Transplantation Research Group of Ile de France. Eur J Med *2*, 339-343.

Fidler, I. J. (1975). Biological behavior of malignant melanoma cells correlated to their survival in vivo. Cancer Res *35*, 218-224.

Flament, H., Alonso Ramirez, R., Premel, V., Joncker, N. T., Jacquet, A., Scholl, S., and Lantz, O. (2015). Modeling the specific CD4+ T cell response against a tumor neoantigen. J Immunol *194*, 3501-3512.

Flanagan, S. P. (1966). 'Nude', a new hairless gene with pleiotropic effects in the mouse. Genet Res *8*, 295-309.

Flood, P. M., Urban, J. L., Kripke, M. L., and Schreiber, H. (1981). Loss of tumor-specific and idiotype-specific immunity with age. J Exp Med *154*, 275-290.

Freedman, A. S., Freeman, G. J., Rhynhart, K., and Nadler, L. M. (1991). Selective induction of B7/BB-1 on interferon-gamma stimulated monocytes: a potential mechanism for amplification of T cell activation through the CD28 pathway. Cell Immunol *137*, 429-437.

Frese, K. K., and Tuveson, D. A. (2007). Maximizing mouse cancer models. Nat Rev Cancer *7*, 645-658.

Fridman, W. H., Pages, F., Sautes-Fridman, C., and Galon, J. (2012). The immune contexture in human tumours: impact on clinical outcome. Nat Rev Cancer *12*, 298-306.

Frisch, S. M., and Francis, H. (1994). Disruption of epithelial cell-matrix interactions induces apoptosis. J Cell Biol *124*, 619-626.

Gajewski, T. F., Schreiber, H., and Fu, Y. X. (2013). Innate and adaptive immune cells in the tumor microenvironment. Nat Immunol *14*, 1014-1022.

Galon, J., Costes, A., Sanchez-Cabo, F., Kirilovsky, A., Mlecnik, B., Lagorce-Pages, C., Tosolini, M., Camus, M., Berger, A., Wind, P., *et al.* (2006). Type, density, and location of immune cells within human colorectal tumors predict clinical outcome. Science *313*, 1960-1964.

Gao, F. G., Khammanivong, V., Liu, W. J., Leggatt, G. R., Frazer, I. H., and Fernando, G. J. (2002). Antigen-specific CD4+ T-cell help is required to activate a memory CD8+ T cell to a fully functional tumor killer cell. Cancer Res *62*, 6438-6441.

Gossen, M., and Bujard, H. (1992). Tight control of gene expression in mammalian cells by tetracycline-responsive promoters. Proceedings of the National Academy of Sciences *89*, 5547-5551.

Gotter, J., Brors, B., Hergenhahn, M., and Kyewski, B. (2004). Medullary epithelial cells of the human thymus express a highly diverse selection of tissue-specific genes colocalized in chromosomal clusters. J Exp Med *199*, 155-166.

Grant, G. A., and Miller, J. F. (1965). Effect of neonatal thymectomy on the induction of sarcomata in C57 BL mice. Nature *205*, 1124-1125.

Greenberg, N. M., DeMayo, F., Finegold, M. J., Medina, D., Tilley, W. D., Aspinall, J. O., Cunha, G. R., Donjacour, A. A., Matusik, R. J., and Rosen, J. M. (1995). Prostate cancer in a transgenic mouse. Proceedings of the National Academy of Sciences *92*, 3439-3443.

Greenberg, P. D., Cheever, M. A., and Fefer, A. (1981). Eradication of disseminated murine leukemia by chemoimmunotherapy with cyclophosphamide and adoptively transferred immune syngeneic Lyt-1+2-lymphocytes. J Exp Med *154*, 952-963.

Gros, A., Parkhurst, M. R., Tran, E., Pasetto, A., Robbins, P. F., Ilyas, S., Prickett, T. D., Gartner, J. J., Crystal, J. S., Roberts, I. M., *et al.* (2016). Prospective identification of neoantigen-specific lymphocytes in the peripheral blood of melanoma patients. Nat Med *22*, 433-438.

Grulich, A. E., van Leeuwen, M. T., Falster, M. O., and Vajdic, C. M. (2007). Incidence of cancers in people with HIV/AIDS compared with immunosuppressed transplant recipients: a meta-analysis. Lancet *370*, 59-67.

Guidoboni, M., Gafa, R., Viel, A., Doglioni, C., Russo, A., Santini, A., Del Tin, L., Macri, E., Lanza, G., Boiocchi, M., and Dolcetti, R. (2001). Microsatellite instability and high content of activated cytotoxic lymphocytes identify colon cancer patients with a favorable prognosis. Am J Pathol *159*, 297-304.

Hahn, W. C., and Weinberg, R. A. (2002). Rules for making human tumor cells. N Engl J Med *347*, 1593-1603.

Hanahan, D. (1985). Heritable formation of pancreatic β-cell tumours in transgenic mice expressing recombinant insulin/simian virus 40 oncogenes. Nature *315*, 115-122.

Hanson, H. L., Donermeyer, D. L., Ikeda, H., White, J. M., Shankaran, V., Old, L. J., Shiku, H., Schreiber, R. D., and Allen, P. M. (2000). Eradication of established tumors by CD8+ T cell adoptive immunotherapy. Immunity *13*, 265-276.

Haverkos, H. W., and Drotman, D. P. (1985). Prevalence of Kaposi's sarcoma among patients with AIDS. N Engl J Med *312*, 1518.

Heath, W. R., Belz, G. T., Behrens, G. M., Smith, C. M., Forehan, S. P., Parish, I. A., Davey, G. M., Wilson, N. S., Carbone, F. R., and Villadangos, J. A. (2004). Cross-presentation, dendritic cell subsets, and the generation of immunity to cellular antigens. Immunol Rev *199*, 9-26.

Hill, G. J., 2nd, and Littlejohn, K. (1971). B16 melanoma in C57BL-6J mice: kinetics and effects of heterologous serum. J Surg Oncol *3*, 1-7.

Hinds, P., and Pietruska, J. (2017). Senescence and tumor suppression. F1000Res *6*, 2121.

Hogquist, K. A., Jameson, S. C., Heath, W. R., Howard, J. L., Bevan, M. J., and Carbone, F. R. (1994). T cell receptor antagonist peptides induce positive selection. Cell *76*, 17-27.

Huang, A. Y., Bruce, A. T., Pardoll, D. M., and Levitsky, H. I. (1996). In vivo cross-priming of MHC class I-restricted antigens requires the TAP transporter. Immunity *4*, 349-355.

Huang, A. Y., Golumbek, P., Ahmadzadeh, M., Jaffee, E., Pardoll, D., and Levitsky, H. (1994). Role of bone marrow-derived cells in presenting MHC class I-restricted tumor antigens. Science *264*, 961-965.

Hughes, C. S., Postovit, L. M., and Lajoie, G. A. (2010). Matrigel: a complex protein mixture required for optimal growth of cell culture. Proteomics *10*, 1886-1890.

Institute of Medicine Immunization Safety Review, C. (2002). In Immunization Safety Review: SV40 Contamination of Polio Vaccine and Cancer, K. Stratton, D.A. Almario, and M.C. McCormick, eds. (Washington (DC): National Academies Press (US)

Copyright 2003 by the National Academy of Sciences. All rights reserved.).

Ishikawa, T., Fujita, T., Suzuki, Y., Okabe, S., Yuasa, Y., Iwai, T., and Kawakami, Y. (2003). Tumor-specific immunological recognition of frameshift-mutated peptides in colon cancer with microsatellite instability. Cancer Res *63*, 5564-5572.

Iwasaki, A., and Medzhitov, R. (2015). Control of adaptive immunity by the innate immune system. Nat Immunol *16*, 343-353.

Jaenisch, R., and Mintz, B. (1974). Simian virus 40 DNA sequences in DNA of healthy adult mice derived from preimplantation blastocysts injected with viral DNA. Proc Natl Acad Sci U S A *71*, 1250-1254.

Janeway, C. A., Jr., and Medzhitov, R. (2002). Innate immune recognition. Annu Rev Immunol *20*, 197-216.

Jenkinson, S. R., Williams, N. A., and Morgan, D. J. (2005). The role of intercellular adhesion molecule-1/LFA-1 interactions in the generation of tumor-specific CD8+ T cell responses. J Immunol *174*, 3401-3407.

Johnson, L., Mercer, K., Greenbaum, D., Bronson, R. T., Crowley, D., Tuveson, D. A., and Jacks, T. (2001). Somatic activation of the K-ras oncogene causes early onset lung cancer in mice. Nature *410*, 1111-1116.

Joncker, N. T., Bettini, S., Boulet, D., Guiraud, M., and Guerder, S. (2016). The site of tumor development determines immunogenicity via temporal mobilization of antigen-laden dendritic cells in draining lymph nodes. Eur J Immunol *46*, 609-618.

Jonkers, J., and Berns, A. (2004). Oncogene addiction: sometimes a temporary slavery. Cancer Cell *6*, 535-538.

Kammertoens, T., Qin, Z., Briesemeister, D., Bendelac, A., and Blankenstein, T. (2012). B-cells and IL-4 promote methylcholanthrene-induced carcinogenesis but there is no evidence for a role of T/NKT-cells and their effector molecules (Fas-ligand, TNF-alpha, perforin). Int J Cancer *131*, 1499-1508.

Kammertoens, T., Willebrand, R., Erdmann, B., Li, L., Li, Y., Engels, B., Uckert, W., and Blankenstein, T. (2005). CY15, a malignant histiocytic tumor that is phenotypically similar to immature dendritic cells. Cancer Res *65*, 2560-2564.

Kang, T. W., Yevsa, T., Woller, N., Hoenicke, L., Wuestefeld, T., Dauch, D., Hohmeyer, A., Gereke, M., Rudalska, R., Potapova, A., *et al.* (2011). Senescence surveillance of pre-malignant hepatocytes limits liver cancer development. Nature *479*, 547-551.

Kaplan, D. H., Shankaran, V., Dighe, A. S., Stockert, E., Aguet, M., Old, L. J., and Schreiber, R. D. (1998). Demonstration of an interferon gamma-dependent tumor surveillance system in immunocompetent mice. Proc Natl Acad Sci U S A *95*, 7556-7561.

Kastan, M. B., Onyekwere, O., Sidransky, D., Vogelstein, B., and Craig, R. W. (1991). Participation of p53 protein in the cellular response to DNA damage. Cancer Res *51*, 6304-6311.

Kawakami, Y., Eliyahu, S., Delgado, C. H., Robbins, P. F., Rivoltini, L., Topalian, S. L., Miki, T., and Rosenberg, S. A. (1994). Cloning of the gene coding for a shared human melanoma antigen recognized by autologous T cells infiltrating into tumor. Proc Natl Acad Sci U S A *91*, 3515-3519.

Keene, J., and Forman, J. (1982). Helper activity is required for the in vivo generation of cytotoxic T lymphocytes. Journal of Experimental Medicine *155*, 768-782.

Kessler, J. H., Bres-Vloemans, S. A., van Veelen, P. A., de Ru, A., Huijbers, I. J., Camps, M., Mulder, A., Offringa, R., Drijfhout, J. W., Leeksma, O. C., *et al.* (2006). BCR-ABL fusion regions as a source of multiple leukemia-specific CD8+ T-cell epitopes. Leukemia *20*, 1738-1750.

Khong, H. T., and Restifo, N. P. (2002). Natural selection of tumor variants in the generation of "tumor escape" phenotypes. Nat Immunol *3*, 999-1005.

Kim, M. S., Yeon, J. H., and Park, J. K. (2007). A microfluidic platform for 3-dimensional cell culture and cell-based assays. Biomed Microdevices *9*, 25-34.

Kirberg, J., von Boehmer, H., Brocker, T., Rodewald, H. R., and Takeda, S. (2001). Class II essential for CD4 survival. Nat Immunol *2*, 136-137.

Kleijmeer, M. J., Kelly, A., Geuze, H. J., Slot, J. W., Townsend, A., and Trowsdale, J. (1992). Location of MHC-encoded transporters in the endoplasmic reticulum and cis-Golgi. Nature *357*, 342-344.

Klein, C. A. (2009). Parallel progression of primary tumours and metastases. Nat Rev Cancer *9*, 302-312.

Klein, G., and Klein, E. (1977). Immune surveillance against virus-induced tumors and nonrejectability of spontaneous tumors: contrasting consequences of host versus tumor evolution. Proc Natl Acad Sci U S A *74*, 2121-2125.

Klein, G., Sjogren, H. O., Klein, E., and Hellstrom, K. E. (1960). Demonstration of resistance against methylcholanthrene-induced sarcomas in the primary autochthonous host. Cancer Res *20*, 1561-1572.

Kleinman, H. K., and Martin, G. R. (2005). Matrigel: basement membrane matrix with biological activity. Semin Cancer Biol *15*, 378-386.

Kleinman, H. K., McGarvey, M. L., Hassell, J. R., Star, V. L., Cannon, F. B., Laurie, G. W., and Martin, G. R. (1986). Basement membrane complexes with biological activity. Biochemistry *25*, 312-318.

Kripke, M. L. (1974). Antigenicity of murine skin tumors induced by ultraviolet light. J Natl Cancer Inst *53*, 1333-1336.

Kuilman, T., Michaloglou, C., Mooi, W. J., and Peeper, D. S. (2010). The essence of senescence. Genes Dev *24*, 2463-2479.

Kündig, T. M., Bachmann, M. F., DiPaolo, C., Simard, J. J., Battegay, M., Lother, H., Gessner, A., Kuhlcke, K., Ohashi, P. S., Hengartner, H., and et al. (1995). Fibroblasts as efficient antigen-presenting cells in lymphoid organs. Science *268*, 1343-1347.

Kündig, T. M., Shahinian, A., Kawai, K., Mittrucker, H. W., Sebzda, E., Bachmann, M. F., Mak, T. W., and Ohashi, P. S. (1996). Duration of TCR stimulation determines costimulatory requirement of T cells. Immunity *5*, 41-52.

Lane, D. P., and Crawford, L. V. (1979). T antigen is bound to a host protein in SV40-transformed cells. Nature *278*, 261-263.

Leisegang, M., Engels, B., Schreiber, K., Yew, P. Y., Kiyotani, K., Idel, C., Arina, A., Duraiswamy, J., Weichselbaum, R. R., Uckert, W., *et al.* (2016). Eradication of Large Solid Tumors by Gene Therapy with a T-Cell Receptor Targeting a Single Cancer-Specific Point Mutation. Clin Cancer Res *22*, 2734-2743.

Lengauer, C., Kinzler, K. W., and Vogelstein, B. (1998). Genetic instabilities in human cancers. Nature *396*, 643-649.

Limberis, M. P., Bell, C. L., and Wilson, J. M. (2009). Identification of the murine firefly luciferase-specific CD8 T-cell epitopes. Gene Ther *16*, 441-447.

Linsley, P. S., Brady, W., Grosmaire, L., Aruffo, A., Damle, N. K., and Ledbetter, J. A. (1991). Binding of the B cell activation antigen B7 to CD28 costimulates T cell proliferation and interleukin 2 mRNA accumulation. J Exp Med *173*, 721-730.

Linzer, D. I., and Levine, A. J. (1979). Characterization of a 54K dalton cellular SV40 tumor antigen present in SV40-transformed cells and uninfected embryonal carcinoma cells. Cell *17*, 43-52.

Liu, P., Zhang, H., McLellan, A., Vogel, H., and Bradley, A. (1998). Embryonic lethality and tumorigenesis caused by segmental aneuploidy on mouse chromosome 11. Genetics *150*, 1155-1168.

Lu, B. J., Lai, M., Cheng, L., Xu, J. Y., and Huang, Q. (2004). Gastric medullary carcinoma, a distinct entity associated with microsatellite instability-H, prominent intraepithelial lymphocytes and improved prognosis. Histopathology *45*, 485-492.

Lu, P., Weaver, V. M., and Werb, Z. (2012). The extracellular matrix: a dynamic niche in cancer progression. J Cell Biol *196*, 395-406.

Lustgarten, J., Dominguez, A. L., and Thoman, M. (2004). Aged mice develop protective antitumor immune responses with appropriate costimulation. J Immunol *173*, 4510-4515.

Lyman, M. A., Aung, S., Biggs, J. A., and Sherman, L. A. (2004). A spontaneously arising pancreatic tumor does not promote the differentiation of naive CD8+ T lymphocytes into effector CTL. J Immunol *172*, 6558-6567.

Maby, P., Galon, J., and Latouche, J. B. (2016). Frameshift mutations, neoantigens and tumor-specific CD8(+) T cells in microsatellite unstable colorectal cancers. Oncoimmunology *5*, e1115943.

Maby, P., Tougeron, D., Hamieh, M., Mlecnik, B., Kora, H., Bindea, G., Angell, H. K., Fredriksen, T., Elie, N., Fauquembergue, E., *et al.* (2015). Correlation between Density of CD8+ T-cell Infiltrate in Microsatellite Unstable Colorectal Cancers and Frameshift Mutations: A Rationale for Personalized Immunotherapy. Cancer Res *75*, 3446-3455.

Magdaleno, S. M., Wang, G., Mireles, V. L., Ray, M. K., Finegold, M. J., and DeMayo, F. J. (1997). Cyclin-dependent kinase inhibitor expression in pulmonary Clara cells transformed with SV40 large T antigen in transgenic mice. Cell growth & differentiation: the molecular biology journal of the American Association for Cancer Research *8*, 145-155.

Maletzki, C., Schmidt, F., Dirks, W. G., Schmitt, M., and Linnebacher, M. (2013). Frameshift-derived neoantigens constitute immunotherapeutic targets for patients with microsatellite-instable haematological malignancies: frameshift peptides for treating MSI+ blood cancers. Eur J Cancer *49*, 2587-2595.

Mantovani, A., Allavena, P., Sica, A., and Balkwill, F. (2008). Cancer-related inflammation. Nature *454*, 436.

Martinez-Lostao, L., Anel, A., and Pardo, J. (2015). How Do Cytotoxic Lymphocytes Kill Cancer Cells? Clin Cancer Res *21*, 5047-5056.

Matsushita, H., Vesely, M. D., Koboldt, D. C., Rickert, C. G., Uppaluri, R., Magrini, V. J., Arthur, C. D., White, J. M., Chen, Y. S., Shea, L. K., *et al.* (2012). Cancer exome analysis reveals a T-cell-dependent mechanism of cancer immunoediting. Nature *482*, 400-404.

Matzinger, P. (1994). Tolerance, danger, and the extended family. Annu Rev Immunol *12*, 991-1045.

Meuwissen, R., Linn, S. C., van der Valk, M., Mooi, W. J., and Berns, A. (2001). Mouse model for lung tumorigenesis through Cre/lox controlled sporadic activation of the K-Ras oncogene. Oncogene *20*, 6551-6558.

Mezzanotte, L., Que, I., Kaijzel, E., Branchini, B., Roda, A., and Lowik, C. (2011). Sensitive dual color in vivo bioluminescence imaging using a new red codon optimized firefly luciferase and a green click beetle luciferase. PLoS One *6*, e19277.

Mombaerts, P., Iacomini, J., Johnson, R. S., Herrup, K., Tonegawa, S., and Papaioannou, V. E. (1992). RAG-1-deficient mice have no mature B and T lymphocytes. Cell *68*, 869-877.

Monach, P. A., Meredith, S. C., Siegel, C. T., and Schreiber, H. (1995). A unique tumor antigen produced by a single amino acid substitution. Immunity *2*, 45-59.

Moreau, R., Dausset, J., Bernard, J., and Moullec, J. (1957). [Acquired hemolytic anemia with polyagglutinability of erythrocytes by a new factor present in normal blood]. Bull Mem Soc Med Hop Paris *73*, 569-587.

Morgan, D. J., Kreuwel, H. T., and Sherman, L. A. (1999). Antigen concentration and precursor frequency determine the rate of CD8+ T cell tolerance to peripherally expressed antigens. J Immunol *163*, 723-727.

Morgan, D. J., Liblau, R., Scott, B., Fleck, S., McDevitt, H. O., Sarvetnick, N., Lo, D., and Sherman, L. A. (1996). CD8(+) T cell-mediated spontaneous diabetes in neonatal mice. J Immunol *157*, 978-983.

Mumberg, D., Monach, P. A., Wanderling, S., Philip, M., Toledano, A. Y., Schreiber, R. D., and Schreiber, H. (1999). CD4(+) T cells eliminate MHC class II-negative cancer cells in vivo by indirect effects of IFN-gamma. Proc Natl Acad Sci U S A *96*, 8633-8638.

Murali-Krishna, K., Lau, L. L., Sambhara, S., Lemonnier, F., Altman, J., and Ahmed, R. (1999). Persistence of memory CD8 T cells in MHC class I-deficient mice. Science *286*, 1377-1381.

Murphy, K., Travers, P., and Walport, M. (2008a). Antigen recognition by T cells. In Janeway's Immunobiology, (Garland Science, Taylor & Francis Group, LLC), pp. 123-132.

Murphy, K., Travers, P., and Walport, M. (2008b). T cell-mediated cytotoxicity. In Janeway's Immunobiology, (Garland Science, Taylor & Francis Group, LLC), pp. 364-368.

Mylin, L. M., Bonneau, R. H., Lippolis, J. D., and Tevethia, S. S. (1995). Hierarchy among multiple H-2b-restricted cytotoxic T-lymphocyte epitopes within simian virus 40 T antigen. J Virol *69*, 6665-6677.

Mylin, L. M., Schell, T. D., Roberts, D., Epler, M., Boesteanu, A., Collins, E. J., Frelinger, J. A., Joyce, S., and Tevethia, S. S. (2000). Quantitation of CD8(+) T-lymphocyte responses to multiple epitopes from simian virus 40 (SV40) large T antigen in C57BL/6 mice immunized with SV40, SV40 T-antigen-transformed cells, or vaccinia virus recombinants expressing full-length T antigen or epitope minigenes. J Virol *74*, 6922-6934.

Nakanishi, Y., Pei, X. H., Takayama, K., Bai, F., Izumi, M., Kimotsuki, K., Inoue, K., Minami, T., Wataya, H., and Hara, N. (2000). Polycyclic aromatic hydrocarbon carcinogens increase ubiquitination of p21 protein after the stabilization of p53 and the expression of p21. Am J Respir Cell Mol Biol *22*, 747-754.

Nakata, B., Wang, Y. Q., Yashiro, M., Nishioka, N., Tanaka, H., Ohira, M., Ishikawa, T., Nishino, H., and Hirakawa, K. (2002). Prognostic value of microsatellite instability in resectable pancreatic cancer. Clin Cancer Res *8*, 2536-2540.

Nguyen, L. T., Elford, A. R., Murakami, K., Garza, K. M., Schoenberger, S. P., Odermatt, B., Speiser, D. E., and Ohashi, P. S. (2002). Tumor growth enhances cross-presentation leading to limited T cell activation without tolerance. J Exp Med *195*, 423-435.

Noguchi, Y., Jungbluth, A., Richards, E. C., and Old, L. J. (1996). Effect of interleukin 12 on tumor induction by 3-methylcholanthrene. Proc Natl Acad Sci U S A *93*, 11798-11801.

Nomoto, K., and Takeya, K. (1969). Immunologic properties of methylcholanthrene-induced sarcomas of neonatally thymectomized mice. J Natl Cancer Inst *42*, 445-453.

Ochsenbein, A. F., Sierro, S., Odermatt, B., Pericin, M., Karrer, U., Hermans, J., Hemmi, S., Hengartner, H., and Zinkernagel, R. M. (2001). Roles of tumour localization, second signals and cross priming in cytotoxic T-cell induction. Nature *411*, 1058-1064.

Oertel, S. H., and Riess, H. (2002). Immunosurveillance, immunodeficiency and lymphoproliferations. Recent Results Cancer Res *159*, 1-8.

Offringa, R. (2009). Antigen choice in adoptive T-cell therapy of cancer. Curr Opin Immunol *21*, 190-199.

Ohl, L., Mohaupt, M., Czeloth, N., Hintzen, G., Kiafard, Z., Zwirner, J., Blankenstein, T., Henning, G., and Forster, R. (2004). CCR7 governs skin dendritic cell migration under inflammatory and steady-state conditions. Immunity *21*, 279-288.

Old, L. J., Boyse, E. A., Clarke, D. A., and Carswell, E. A. (1962). Antigenic properties of chemically induced tumors. Annals of the New York Academy of Sciences *101*, 80-106.

Onizuka, S., Tawara, I., Shimizu, J., Sakaguchi, S., Fujita, T., and Nakayama, E. (1999). Tumor rejection by in vivo administration of anti-CD25 (interleukin-2 receptor alpha) monoclonal antibody. Cancer Res *59*, 3128-3133.

Orkin, R. W., Gehron, P., McGoodwin, E. B., Martin, G. R., Valentine, T., and Swarm, R. (1977). A murine tumor producing a matrix of basement membrane. J Exp Med *145*, 204-220.

Otahal, P., Hutchinson, S. C., Mylin, L. M., Tevethia, M. J., Tevethia, S. S., and Schell, T. D. (2005). Inefficient cross-presentation limits the CD8+ T cell response to a subdominant tumor antigen epitope. J Immunol *175*, 700-712.

Pamer, E., and Cresswell, P. (1998). Mechanisms of MHC class I--restricted antigen processing. Annu Rev Immunol *16*, 323-358.

Pardigon, N., Bercovici, N., Calbo, S., Santos-Lima, E. C., Liblau, R., Kourilsky, P., and Abastado, J. P. (1998). Role of co-stimulation in CD8+ T cell activation. Int Immunol *10*, 619-630.

Pavelic, V., Matter, M. S., Mumprecht, S., Breyer, I., and Ochsenbein, A. F. (2009). CTL induction by cross-priming is restricted to immunodominant epitopes. Eur J Immunol *39*, 704-716.

Pircher, H., Burki, K., Lang, R., Hengartner, H., and Zinkernagel, R. M. (1989). Tolerance induction in double specific T-cell receptor transgenic mice varies with antigen. Nature *342*, 559-561.

Plattner, B. L., Huffman, E. L., and Hostetter, J. M. (2013). Gamma-delta T-cell responses during subcutaneous Mycobacterium avium subspecies paratuberculosis challenge in sensitized or naive calves using matrix biopolymers. Vet Pathol *50*, 630-637.

Prehn, R. T., and Main, J. M. (1957). Immunity to methylcholanthrene-induced sarcomas. J Natl Cancer Inst *18*, 769-778.

Qin, Z., and Blankenstein, T. (2000). CD4+ T cell--mediated tumor rejection involves inhibition of angiogenesis that is dependent on IFN gamma receptor expression by nonhematopoietic cells. Immunity *12*, 677-686.

Qin, Z., and Blankenstein, T. (2004). A cancer immunosurveillance controversy. Nat Immunol *5*, 3-4; author reply 4-5.

Quezada, S. A., Simpson, T. R., Peggs, K. S., Merghoub, T., Vider, J., Fan, X., Blasberg, R., Yagita, H., Muranski, P., Antony, P. A., *et al.* (2010). Tumor-reactive CD4(+) T cells develop cytotoxic activity and eradicate large established melanoma after transfer into lymphopenic hosts. J Exp Med *207*, 637-650.

Reuschenbach, M., Kloor, M., Morak, M., Wentzensen, N., Germann, A., Garbe, Y., Tariverdian, M., Findeisen, P., Neumaier, M., Holinski-Feder, E., and von Knebel Doeberitz, M. (2010). Serum antibodies against frameshift peptides in microsatellite unstable colorectal cancer patients with Lynch syndrome. Fam Cancer *9*, 173-179.

Rice, B. W., Cable, M. D., and Nelson, M. B. (2001). In vivo imaging of light-emitting probes. J Biomed Opt *6*, 432-440.

Rizzuto, G. A., Merghoub, T., Hirschhorn-Cymerman, D., Liu, C., Lesokhin, A. M., Sahawneh, D., Zhong, H., Panageas, K. S., Perales, M. A., Altan-Bonnet, G., et al. (2009). Self-antigen-specific CD8+ T cell precursor frequency determines the quality of the antitumor immune response. J Exp Med *206*, 849-866.

Robbins, P. F., Lu, Y. C., El-Gamil, M., Li, Y. F., Gross, C., Gartner, J., Lin, J. C., Teer, J. K., Cliften, P., Tycksen, E., et al. (2013). Mining exomic sequencing data to identify mutated antigens recognized by adoptively transferred tumor-reactive T cells. Nat Med *19*, 747-752.

Rodier, F., and Campisi, J. (2011). Four faces of cellular senescence. J Cell Biol *192*, 547-556.

Rodriguez, A., Regnault, A., Kleijmeer, M., Ricciardi-Castagnoli, P., and Amigorena, S. (1999). Selective transport of internalized antigens to the cytosol for MHC class I presentation in dendritic cells. Nat Cell Biol *1*, 362-368.

Ryan, M. H., Bristol, J. A., McDuffie, E., and Abrams, S. I. (2001). Regression of extensive pulmonary metastases in mice by adoptive transfer of antigen-specific CD8(+) CTL reactive against tumor cells expressing a naturally occurring rejection epitope. J Immunol *167*, 4286-4292.

Saenz-Robles, M. T., Sullivan, C. S., and Pipas, J. M. (2001). Transforming functions of Simian Virus 40. Oncogene *20*, 7899-7907.

Saeterdal, I., Bjorheim, J., Lislerud, K., Gjertsen, M. K., Bukholm, I. K., Olsen, O. C., Nesland, J. M., Eriksen, J. A., Moller, M., Lindblom, A., and Gaudernack, G. (2001). Frameshift-mutation-derived peptides as tumor-specific antigens in inherited and spontaneous colorectal cancer. Proc Natl Acad Sci U S A *98*, 13255-13260.

Sakaguchi, S., Miyara, M., Costantino, C. M., and Hafler, D. A. (2010). FOXP3+ regulatory T cells in the human immune system. Nat Rev Immunol *10*, 490-500.

Savage, P. A., Vosseller, K., Kang, C., Larimore, K., Riedel, E., Wojnoonski, K., Jungbluth, A. A., and Allison, J. P. (2008). Recognition of a ubiquitous self antigen by prostate cancer-infiltrating CD8+ T lymphocytes. Science *319*, 215-220.

Scanlan, M. J., Gure, A. O., Jungbluth, A. A., Old, L. J., and Chen, Y. T. (2002). Cancer/testis antigens: an expanding family of targets for cancer immunotherapy. Immunol Rev *188*, 22-32.

Schietinger, A., Arina, A., Liu, R. B., Wells, S., Huang, J., Engels, B., Bindokas, V., Bartkowiak, T., Lee, D., Herrmann, A., et al. (2013). Longitudinal confocal microscopy imaging of solid tumor destruction following adoptive T cell transfer. Oncoimmunology *2*, e26677.

Schietinger, A., Philip, M., Yoshida, B. A., Azadi, P., Liu, H., Meredith, S. C., and Schreiber, H. (2006). A mutant chaperone converts a wild-type protein into a tumor-specific antigen. Science *314*, 304-308.

Schreiber, H. (2012a). Cancer immunology. In Fundamentals of Immunology, W.E. Paul, ed. (Lippincott Williams&Wilki), p. 1207.

Schreiber, H. (2012b). Cancer Immunology. In Fundamental Immunology, W.E. Paul, ed. (Lippincott, Williams & Wilkins), pp. 1223-1225.

Schreiber, K., Arina, A., Engels, B., Spiotto, M. T., Sidney, J., Sette, A., Karrison, T. G., Weichselbaum, R. R., Rowley, D. A., and Schreiber, H. (2012). Spleen cells from young but not old immunized mice eradicate large established cancers. Clin Cancer Res *18*, 2526-2533.

Schreiber, K., Rowley, D. A., Riethmuller, G., and Schreiber, H. (2006). Cancer immunotherapy and preclinical studies: why we are not wasting our time with animal experiments. Hematol Oncol Clin North Am *20*, 567-584.

Schreiber, T. H., and Podack, E. R. (2009). A critical analysis of the tumour immunosurveillance controversy for 3-MCA-induced sarcomas. Br J Cancer *101*, 381-386.

Schwartz, R. H. (1990). A cell culture model for T lymphocyte clonal anergy. Science *248*, 1349-1356.

Schwartz, R. H. (2003). T cell anergy. Annu Rev Immunol *21*, 305-334.

Shankaran, V., Ikeda, H., Bruce, A. T., White, J. M., Swanson, P. E., Old, L. J., and Schreiber, R. D. (2001). IFNgamma and lymphocytes prevent primary tumour development and shape tumour immunogenicity. Nature *410*, 1107-1111.

Shen, F. W., Saga, Y., Litman, G., Freeman, G., Tung, J. S., Cantor, H., and Boyse, E. A. (1985). Cloning of Ly-5 cDNA. Proc Natl Acad Sci U S A *82*, 7360-7363.

Shimizu, J., Yamazaki, S., and Sakaguchi, S. (1999). Induction of tumor immunity by removing CD25+CD4+ T cells: a common basis between tumor immunity and autoimmunity. J Immunol *163*, 5211-5218.

Simoni, Y., Becht, E., Fehlings, M., Loh, C. Y., Koo, S. L., Teng, K. W. W., Yeong, J. P. S., Nahar, R., Zhang, T., Kared, H., *et al.* (2018). Bystander CD8(+) T cells are abundant and phenotypically distinct in human tumour infiltrates. Nature *557*, 575-579.

Simpson, A. J., Caballero, O. L., Jungbluth, A., Chen, Y. T., and Old, L. J. (2005). Cancer/testis antigens, gametogenesis and cancer. Nat Rev Cancer *5*, 615-625.

Smyth, M. J., Thia, K. Y., Cretney, E., Kelly, J. M., Snook, M. B., Forbes, C. A., and Scalzo, A. A. (1999). Perforin is a major contributor to NK cell control of tumor metastasis. J Immunol *162*, 6658-6662.

Speiser, D. E., Miranda, R., Zakarian, A., Bachmann, M. F., McKall-Faienza, K., Odermatt, B., Hanahan, D., Zinkernagel, R. M., and Ohashi, P. S. (1997). Self antigens expressed by solid tumors Do not efficiently stimulate naive or activated T cells: implications for immunotherapy. J Exp Med *186*, 645-653.

Spellman, C. W., and Daynes, R. A. (1978). Immunoregulation by ultraviolet light-III. Enhancement of suppressor cell activity in older animals. Exp Gerontol *13*, 141-146.

Spiotto, M. T., Reth, M. A., and Schreiber, H. (2003). Genetic changes occurring in established tumors rapidly stimulate new antibody responses. Proc Natl Acad Sci U S A *100*, 5425-5430.

Spiotto, M. T., Yu, P., Rowley, D. A., Nishimura, M. I., Meredith, S. C., Gajewski, T. F., Fu, Y. X., and Schreiber, H. (2002). Increasing tumor antigen expression overcomes "ignorance" to solid tumors via crosspresentation by bone marrow-derived stromal cells. Immunity *17*, 737-747.

Staveley-O'Carroll, K., Schell, T. D., Jimenez, M., Mylin, L. M., Tevethia, M. J., Schoenberger, S. P., and Tevethia, S. S. (2003). In vivo ligation of CD40 enhances priming against the endogenous tumor antigen and promotes CD8+ T cell effector function in SV40 T antigen transgenic mice. J Immunol *171*, 697-707.

Stewart, N., and Bacchetti, S. (1991). Expression of SV40 large T antigen, but not small t antigen, is required for the induction of chromosomal aberrations in transformed human cells. Virology *180*, 49-57.

Stutman, O. (1974). Tumor development after 3-methylcholanthrene in immunologically deficient athymic-nude mice. Science *183*, 534-536.

Swann, J. B., Vesely, M. D., Silva, A., Sharkey, J., Akira, S., Schreiber, R. D., and Smyth, M. J. (2008). Demonstration of inflammation-induced cancer and cancer immunoediting during primary tumorigenesis. Proc Natl Acad Sci U S A *105*, 652-656.

Szyska, M., Herda, S., Althoff, S., Heimann, A., Russ, J., D'Abundo, D., Dang, T. M., Durieux, I., Dorken, B., Blankenstein, T., and Na, I. K. (2018). A Transgenic Dual-Luciferase Reporter Mouse for Longitudinal and Functional Monitoring of T Cells In Vivo. Cancer Immunol Res 6, 110-120.

Takahashi, T., Nau, M. M., Chiba, I., Birrer, M. J., Rosenberg, R. K., Vinocour, M., Levitt, M., Pass, H., Gazdar, A. F., and Minna, J. D. (1989). p53: a frequent target for genetic abnormalities in lung cancer. Science 246, 491-494.

Tanaka, H., Arakawa, H., Yamaguchi, T., Shiraishi, K., Fukuda, S., Matsui, K., Takei, Y., and Nakamura, Y. (2000). A ribonucleotide reductase gene involved in a p53-dependent cell-cycle checkpoint for DNA damage. Nature 404, 42-49.

Tanchot, C., Lemonnier, F. A., Perarnau, B., Freitas, A. A., and Rocha, B. (1997a). Differential requirements for survival and proliferation of CD8 naive or memory T cells. Science 276, 2057-2062.

Tanchot, C., Rosado, M. M., Agenes, F., Freitas, A. A., and Rocha, B. (1997b). Lymphocyte homeostasis. Semin Immunol 9, 331-337.

Tempero, R. M., VanLith, M. L., Morikane, K., Rowse, G. J., Gendler, S. J., and Hollingsworth, M. A. (1998). CD4+ lymphocytes provide MUC1-specific tumor immunity in vivo that is undetectable in vitro and is absent in MUC1 transgenic mice. J Immunol 161, 5500-5506.

Tevethia, M. J., Bonneau, R. H., Griffith, J. W., and Mylin, L. (1997). A simian virus 40 large T-antigen segment containing amino acids 1 to 127 and expressed under the control of the rat elastase-1 promoter produces pancreatic acinar carcinomas in transgenic mice. J Virol 71, 8157-8166.

Textor, A., Schmidt, K., Kloetzel, P. M., Weissbrich, B., Perez, C., Charo, J., Anders, K., Sidney, J., Sette, A., Schumacher, T. N., et al. (2016). Preventing tumor escape by targeting a post-proteasomal trimming independent epitope. J Exp Med 213, 2333-2348.

Thomas, L. (1959). Cellular and humoral aspects of the hypersensitive states 9, 529-532.

Tong, P. L., Roediger, B., Kolesnikoff, N., Biro, M., Tay, S. S., Jain, R., Shaw, L. E., Grimbaldeston, M. A., and Weninger, W. (2015). The skin immune atlas: three-dimensional analysis of cutaneous leukocyte subsets by multiphoton microscopy. J Invest Dermatol 135, 84-93.

Townsend, A., and Bodmer, H. (1989). Antigen recognition by class I-restricted T lymphocytes. Annu Rev Immunol 7, 601-624.

Tran, E., Turcotte, S., Gros, A., Robbins, P. F., Lu, Y.-C., Dudley, M. E., Wunderlich, J. R., Somerville, R. P., Hogan, K., Hinrichs, C. S., et al. (2014). Cancer Immunotherapy Based on Mutation-Specific CD4+ T Cells in a Patient with Epithelial Cancer. Science 344, 641-645.

Traversari, C., van der Bruggen, P., Luescher, I. F., Lurquin, C., Chomez, P., Van Pel, A., De Plaen, E., Amar-Costesec, A., and Boon, T. (1992). A nonapeptide encoded by human gene MAGE-1 is recognized on HLA-A1 by cytolytic T lymphocytes directed against tumor antigen MZ2-E. J Exp Med 176, 1453-1457.

Troy, T., Jekic-McMullen, D., Sambucetti, L., and Rice, B. (2004). Quantitative comparison of the sensitivity of detection of fluorescent and bioluminescent reporters in animal models. Mol Imaging 3, 9-23.

Uckun, F. M., Jaszcz, W., Ambrus, J. L., Fauci, A. S., Gajl-Peczalska, K., Song, C. W., Wick, M. R., Myers, D. E., Waddick, K., and Ledbetter, J. A. (1988). Detailed studies on expression and function of CD19 surface determinant by using B43 monoclonal antibody and the clinical potential of anti-CD19 immunotoxins. Blood 71, 13-29.

Urlinger, S., Baron, U., Thellmann, M., Hasan, M. T., Bujard, H., and Hillen, W. (2000). Exploring the sequence space for tetracycline-dependent transcriptional activators: novel mutations yield expanded range and sensitivity. Proc Natl Acad Sci U S A 97, 7963-7968.

van den Broek, M. E., Kagi, D., Ossendorp, F., Toes, R., Vamvakas, S., Lutz, W. K., Melief, C. J., Zinkernagel, R. M., and Hengartner, H. (1996). Decreased tumor surveillance in perforin-deficient mice. J Exp Med *184*, 1781-1790.

van Houdt, I. S., Sluijter, B. J., Moesbergen, L. M., Vos, W. M., de Gruijl, T. D., Molenkamp, B. G., van den Eertwegh, A. J., Hooijberg, E., van Leeuwen, P. A., Meijer, C. J., and Oudejans, J. J. (2008). Favorable outcome in clinically stage II melanoma patients is associated with the presence of activated tumor infiltrating T-lymphocytes and preserved MHC class I antigen expression. Int J Cancer *123*, 609-615.

van Mierlo, G. J., Boonman, Z. F., Dumortier, H. M., den Boer, A. T., Fransen, M. F., Nouta, J., van der Voort, E. I., Offringa, R., Toes, R. E., and Melief, C. J. (2004). Activation of dendritic cells that cross-present tumor-derived antigen licenses CD8+ CTL to cause tumor eradication. J Immunol *173*, 6753-6759.

Vitale, M., Rezzani, R., Rodella, L., Zauli, G., Grigolato, P., Cadei, M., Hicklin, D. J., and Ferrone, S. (1998). HLA class I antigen and transporter associated with antigen processing (TAP1 and TAP2) down-regulation in high-grade primary breast carcinoma lesions. Cancer Res *58*, 737-742.

Vogelstein, B., Lane, D., and Levine, A. J. (2000). Surfing the p53 network. Nature *408*, 307-310.

Vukicevic, S., Kleinman, H. K., Luyten, F. P., Roberts, A. B., Roche, N. S., and Reddi, A. H. (1992). Identification of multiple active growth factors in basement membrane Matrigel suggests caution in interpretation of cellular activity related to extracellular matrix components. Exp Cell Res *202*, 1-8.

Ward, P. L., Koeppen, H., Hurteau, T., and Schreiber, H. (1989). Tumor antigens defined by cloned immunological probes are highly polymorphic and are not detected on autologous normal cells. J Exp Med *170*, 217-232.

Weinstein, I. B., and Joe, A. (2008). Oncogene addiction. Cancer Res *68*, 3077-3080; discussion 3080.

Wen, F. T., Thisted, R. A., Rowley, D. A., and Schreiber, H. (2012). A systematic analysis of experimental immunotherapies on tumors differing in size and duration of growth. Oncoimmunology *1*, 172-178.

Willimsky, G., and Blankenstein, T. (2005). Sporadic immunogenic tumours avoid destruction by inducing T-cell tolerance. Nature *437*, 141-146.

Willimsky, G., Czeh, M., Loddenkemper, C., Gellermann, J., Schmidt, K., Wust, P., Stein, H., and Blankenstein, T. (2008). Immunogenicity of premalignant lesions is the primary cause of general cytotoxic T lymphocyte unresponsiveness. J Exp Med *205*, 1687-1700.

Willimsky, G., Schmidt, K., Loddenkemper, C., Gellermann, J., and Blankenstein, T. (2013). Virus-induced hepatocellular carcinomas cause antigen-specific local tolerance. J Clin Invest *123*, 1032-1043.

Wilson, T., and Hastings, J. W. (1998). Bioluminescence. Annu Rev Cell Dev Biol *14*, 197-230.

Wolfel, T., Hauer, M., Schneider, J., Serrano, M., Wolfel, C., Klehmann-Hieb, E., De Plaen, E., Hankeln, T., Meyer zum Buschenfelde, K. H., and Beach, D. (1995). A p16INK4a-insensitive CDK4 mutant targeted by cytolytic T lymphocytes in a human melanoma. Science *269*, 1281-1284.

Wolkers, M. C., Stoetter, G., Vyth-Dreese, F. A., and Schumacher, T. N. (2001). Redundancy of direct priming and cross-priming in tumor-specific CD8+ T cell responses. J Immunol *167*, 3577-3584.

Xiong, Y., Hannon, G. J., Zhang, H., Casso, D., Kobayashi, R., and Beach, D. (1993). p21 is a universal inhibitor of cyclin kinases. Nature *366*, 701-704.

Yewdell, J. W., and Bennink, J. R. (1992). Cell biology of antigen processing and presentation to major histocompatibility complex class I molecule-restricted T lymphocytes. In Advances in immunology, (Elsevier), pp. 1-123.

Yewdell, J. W., Esquivel, F., Arnold, D., Spies, T., Eisenlohr, L. C., and Bennink, J. R. (1993). Presentation of numerous viral peptides to mouse major histocompatibility complex (MHC) class I-restricted T lymphocytes is mediated by the human MHC-encoded transporter or by a hybrid mouse-human transporter. J Exp Med *177*, 1785-1790.

Yonish-Rouach, E., Resnitzky, D., Lotem, J., Sachs, L., Kimchi, A., and Oren, M. (1991). Wild-type p53 induces apoptosis of myeloid leukaemic cells that is inhibited by interleukin-6. Nature *352*, 345-347.

You, L., Mao, L., Wei, J., Jin, S., Yang, C., Liu, H., Zhu, L., and Qian, W. (2017). The crosstalk between autophagic and endo-/exosomal pathways in antigen processing for MHC presentation in anticancer T cell immune responses. J Hematol Oncol *10*, 165.

Yu, P., Spiotto, M. T., Lee, Y., Schreiber, H., and Fu, Y. X. (2003). Complementary role of CD4+ T cells and secondary lymphoid tissues for cross-presentation of tumor antigen to CD8+ T cells. J Exp Med *197*, 985-995.

Zaid, A., Mackay, L. K., Rahimpour, A., Braun, A., Veldhoen, M., Carbone, F. R., Manton, J. H., Heath, W. R., and Mueller, S. N. (2014). Persistence of skin-resident memory T cells within an epidermal niche. Proc Natl Acad Sci U S A *111*, 5307-5312.

Zhang, L., Conejo-Garcia, J. R., Katsaros, D., Gimotty, P. A., Massobrio, M., Regnani, G., Makrigiannakis, A., Gray, H., Schlienger, K., Liebman, M. N., *et al.* (2003). Intratumoral T cells, recurrence, and survival in epithelial ovarian cancer. N Engl J Med *348*, 203-213.

Zhou, Q., Johnson, B. D., and Orentas, R. J. (2007). Cellular immune response to an engineered cell-based tumor vaccine at the vaccination site. Cell Immunol *245*, 91-102.

7 Abbreviations

α	alpha
β	beta
γ	gamma
δ	delta
µl	micro liter
aa	amino acid
as	antisense
ACK	ammonium-chloride-potassium
ACT	adoptive cell transfer
AdCre	adenovirus encoding Cre
AIDS	acquired immune deficiency syndrome
APC	antigen presenting cell
ATT	adoptive T cell transfer
BAX	Bcl-2 associated X protein
BL	bioluminescence
BLI	bioluminescence imaging
bp	base pair
BrdU	5-bromo-2'-deoxyuridine
BV	brilliant violet
CAG	promoter consisting of elements from Cytomegalovirus, beta-Actin and rabbit beta-Globin gene
CAT	chloramphenicol acetyltransferase
CCD	charge-coupled device
CD	cluster of differentiation
CDK	cyclin-dependent kinase
CFSE	carboxyfluorescein succinimidyl ester
CMV	cytomegalovirus
Cre	Cre recombinase
d	day(s)
DNA	deoxyribonucleic acid
DC	dendritic cell
dLN	draining lymph node
dox	doxycycline
EDTA	ethylenediaminetetraacetic acid
e.g.	exempli gratia (for example)
ELISA	enzyme-linked immunosorbent assay
ER	endoplasmic reticulum

FACS	fluorescence-activated cell sorting
FC	flow cytometry
FCS	fetal calf serum
FITC	fluorescein isothiocyanate
Fluc	firefly luciferase
GEMM	genetically engineered mouse model
gp-100	glycoprotein 100
h	hour
HER2	human epidermal growth receptor 2
HHV-8	human herpes virus 8
HIV	human immunodeficiency virus
HRP	horseradish peroxidase
hsc70	heat shock 70 kDa protein 8
ICAM-1	intercellular adhesion molecule 1
IFN-γ	interferon γ
Ig	immunoglobulin
IL	interleukin
i.v.	intravenous, -ly
kb	kilo base
kDa	kilo Dalton
LFA-1	lymphocyte function-associated antigen 1
LN	lymph node
loxP	locus of X-over P1
Luc	luciferase
MACS	magnetic-activated cell sorting
MAGE	melanoma-associated antigen
MART1	melanoma antigen recognized by T cells 1
MCA	3-methylcholanthrene
MFI	mean fluorescence intensity
MHC	major histocompatibility complex
min	minute(s)
ml	milli liter
mRNA	messenger RNA
MSI	microsatellite instability
MUC1	mucin 1
ndLN	non-draining lymph node
NFAT	nuclear factor of activated T cells
NK	natural killer
NKT	nature killer T
p	peptide
PBS	phosphate buffered saline
PCR	polymerase chain reaction

PE	phycoerythrin
pI	peptide I
PI	propidium iodide
pIV	peptide IV
rpm	revolutions per minute
Rb	retinoblastoma
RLU	relative light unit
RNA	ribonucleic acid
rtTA	reverse tetracycline-controlled transcription activator
s	second(s)
SA	senescence-associated
s.c.	subcutaneous, -ly
SD	standard deviation
se	sense
SEM	standard error of the mean
STAT1	signal transducer and activator of transcription 1
SV40	simian virus 40
Tag	SV40 large T
TAP	transporter associated with antigen processing
TC	TRE^{loxP}stop^{loxP}TagLuc x CAG-rtTA
TCR	T cell receptor
Tet	tetracycline
tetO	Tn10 tetracycline-resistant operon
tetR	tetracycline repressor protein
TIL	tumor-infiltrating lymphocyte
TRE	tetracycline-responsive element
T$_{reg}$	regulatory T cell
tTA	tetracycline-controlled transcription activator
TTC	TRE^{loxP}stop^{loxP}TagLuc x CAG-rtTA x TyrCre
UV	ultraviolet
VP16	virion protein 16
WB	western blot
WT-1	Wilms' tumor protein 1

8 Acknowledgement

I would like to thank all those people who made this thesis possible and a unique experience for me.

First, I would like to thank my supervisor Prof. Dr. Thomas Blankenstein for giving me the opportunity to work in his group and for all his support and guidance during the time of research. He provided me this interesting but challenging project and was always open to excellent and rewarding discussions that helped me evolving my scientific mind and developing own ideas.

I would also like to thank all present and former members of the lab of Prof. Dr. Thomas Blankenstein. Special thanks go to Dr. Kathleen Anders, my mentor during my whole doctoral studies. She convinced me to enter the exciting field of tumor immunology and supported me by sharing all her knowledge with great patience and passion. She always had an open ear for all my questions and was available for a coffee break whenever it was needed. She kept a general overview about my project whenever I was lost in the details. Further, I would like to thank Dr. Ana Milojkovic for giving me profound insights into the topic of senescence, but also for cheering me up at our Mensa times. Great thanks go to Isabell Becker, whose technical expertise was imperative in the lab. Her calm, considerate and diligent attitude made working with her very joyful. I would also like to thank Isabell Höft and Marion Rösch for their great help in managing the tremendous number of mice and supporting experiments with their blood collecting skills. Thanks to Lucia Poncette, Meng-Tung Hsu and Arunraj Dhamodaran for always being there for discussions, laughs and breaks.

Finally, I would like to thank my family and friends: My parents, for their support and belief in me and for always encouraging me to give my best. My friends Janina and Jacy, who shared with me the ups and downs of a doctoral student's life by walking the same long way. Finally, my deepest thanks to Paul, for his endless love, encouragement and belief in me.

9 Appendix

Morphological changes of TTC #3055 cancer cells upon TagLuc inactivation

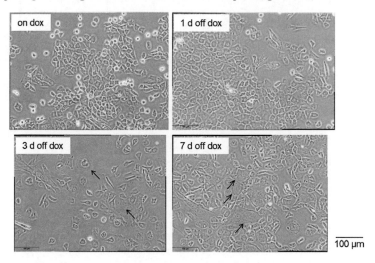

Figure 9.1 Morphological changes of TTC #3055 cancer cells upon TagLuc inactivation
Morphological changes of TTC #3055 cancer cells upon TagLuc inactivation were detected at indicated time
points by phase-contrast light microscopy (40x magnification). 5x10⁵ cancer cells were seeded per well in a
6-well plate and subjected to microscopy at the indicated time points post oncogene inactivation. Black arrows
indicate enlarged and flattened cells with irregular shape.

Clone 3D3 cancer cells

Clone 3D3 cancer cells were derived from clone 4 cancer cells as followed: CM2 mice were
inoculated with clone 4 cancer cells 'off dox' and TagLuc was never induced *in vivo*. Two
months after inoculation, CM2 underwent a tumor challenge with Tet-TagLuc cells which
were subsequently rejected. Unexpectedly, tumors grew out in 2 out of 3 CM2 mice in the
absence of dox/TagLuc induction. Both tumors reached a size of > 1000 mm³ at d 154 post
original clone 4 cancer cell inoculation and a small BL signal was detected that indicated a
low, dox-independent TagLuc expression (Fig. 9.2A). One tumor was isolated, cultured *in
vitro* and tested for dox-mediated TagLuc inducibility. Because TagLuc was still inducible
in the tumor bulk culture (Fig. 9.2A), a single cell cloning in 96-well plate was performed to
obtain a clonal cell line with low TagLuc expression that is still regulated by dox. Among
the generated clones, clone 3D3 showed the required properties: TagLuc was not expressed
in the absence of dox but dox administration induced TagLuc expression at a 250x lower
level than clone 4 cancer cells (Fig. 9.2B).

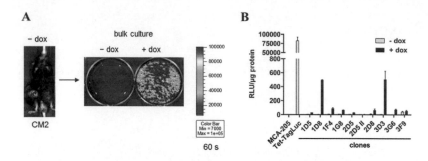

Figure 9.2: Generation of clone 3D3 cancer cells that express low amounts of TagLuc
(A) BL signal of a CM2 mouse that was inoculated with 1×10^5 clone 4 cancer cells 'off dox' (in 10 mg/ml BD Matrigel) 150 d before and which was never administered to dox for TagLuc induction. After culture *in vitro* for few passages and in the absence of dox, 5×10^5 cells were seeded in a 6-well plate, TagLuc was induced via dox (1 μg/ml) and BL signal was measured 3 d later for cells cultured on (+) and off (−) dox. **(B)** Fluc assay was performed with single cell clones derived from cloning of the tumor bulk culture. Clones were grown for 3 d on or off dox, proteins were harvested and subjected to luciferase activity assay. Mean RLU (± SEM) is displayed for each clone. Negative control: MCA-205, positive control: Tet-TagLuc.

Rejection of TagLuc⁺ cancer cells by CD8⁺ T cells in the absence of CD4⁺ T cells

Results from the experiment described in section 3.3.3 were confirmed by a second, independent experiment. Briefly, P14xRag$^{-/-}$ mice were inoculated with 1×10^4 clone 4 cancer cells 'off dox'. TagLuc expression in resting cancer cells was induced by dox 2 weeks post inoculation when the inoculation-induced, acute inflammation was vanished. Simultaneously, mice received 1×10^6 CD8⁺ T cells isolated from the spleen of naïve, young CM2 mice. Splenocyte suspension was either subjected to MACS-depletion of CD4⁺ T cells ('CD4-Φ') or left undepleted ('CD4+CD8') before adoptive transfer.

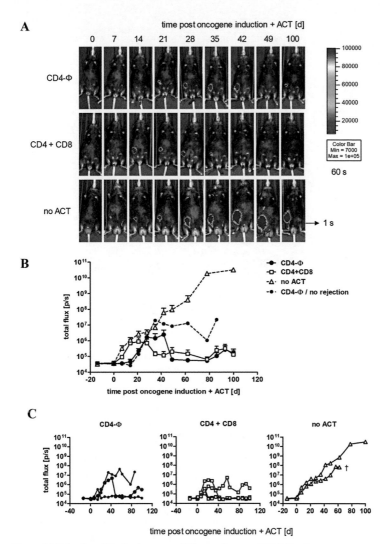

Figure 9.3 Rejection of TagLuc$^+$ cancer cells in the absence of CD4$^+$ T cells

(A) BL signal kinetic of indicated P14xRag$^{-/-}$ mice is shown over time post ACT (d). Each mouse was inoculated with 1x10^4 clone 4 cancer cells 'off dox' (in 10 mg/ml BD Matrigel™). TagLuc was induced by dox administration 14 d post inoculation. Simultaneously, mice received indicated splenocyte suspension derived from CM2 mice and containing 1x10^6 CD8$^+$ T cells i.v. Mice shown are representative for each group (CD4-Φ, n=3; CD4+CD8, n=3; no ACT, n=2). (B) BL signal kinetic over time (in d post ACT) is displayed for each group of mice. Displayed is total flux [p/s] ± SEM. One mouse of group 'CD4-Φ' did not reject clone 4 cancer cells and therefore, it is shown separately (black circle, dashed line). (C) Individual BL signal kinetics of each mouse per group are shown at indicated time point post ACT (d). †, mouse died before end of experiment.

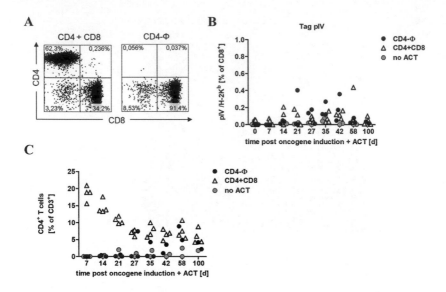

Figure 9.4 Appearance of Tag-specific CD8⁺ T cells and fate of rarely transferred CD4⁺ T cells in P14xRag⁻/⁻ mice after TagLuc induction

(A) Frequency of CD4⁺ T cells in CM2-derived splenocyte suspension either depleted of CD4⁺ T cells ('CD4-Φ') or left untreated ('CD4+CD8') was quantified by flow cytometry. Splenocytes were stained with monoclonal anti-CD3, anti-CD4 and anti-CD8 antibodies. Gate: CD3⁺ lymphocytes. **(B)** Induction of Tag pIV-specific CD8⁺ T cells is displayed over time post ACT (d). Peripheral blood cells were stained with monoclonal anti-CD3 and anti-CD8 antibodies, and P/MHC tetramers loaded with Tag pIV. Frequency of Tag-specific CD8⁺ T cells was analyzed by flow cytometry. CD4-Φ, n=3; CD4+CD8, n=4; no ACT, n=2. **(C)** The fate of transferred CD4⁺ T cells in P14xRag⁻/⁻ mice was followed over time post ACT (d) and is depicted for each mouse. Peripheral blood cells were stained with monoclonal anti-CD3, anti-CD4 and anti-CD8 antibodies and analyzed in a flow cytometer. CD4-Φ, n=3; CD4+CD8, n=4; no ACT, n=2.

The results displayed in Fig. 9.3 and Fig. 9.4. supported the findings obtained from the first experiment described in section 3.3.3 of the presented work. TagLuc-expressing clone 4 cancer cells were rejected in the majority of P14xRag⁻/⁻ mice receiving CD4⁺ T cell depleted splenocytes. In contrast to the first experiment, Tag pIV-specific CD8⁺ T cells expanded less. In some P14xRag⁻/⁻ mice of both groups ('CD4-Φ' and 'CD4+CD8'), no Tag pIV-specific CD8⁺ T cells were detected by flow cytometry despite an observed rejection of the inoculated cancer cells. One reason might be that CD8⁺ T cells expanded only locally at the site were TagLuc was expressed or that contraction of expanded CD8⁺ T cells was within a short time period and thus, missed by the analysis at the indicated days.